LOOK GREAT FEEL GOOD!

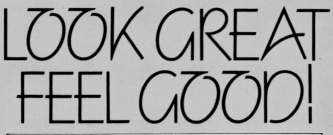

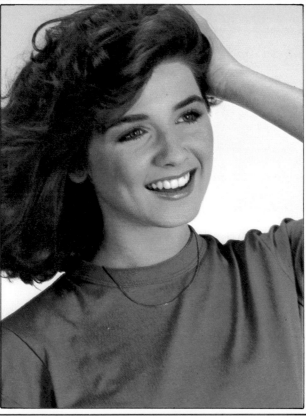

THE COMPLETE GUIDE TO A HEALTHY NEW YOU

Heather Bampfylde

COLLINS

Picture credits

Ambre Solaire: pages 4, 71, 117, 120, 121, 135, 139, 155
Avon Cosmetics Ltd: pages 38, 42, 43, 56, 69
David Bailey reproduced by courtesy of Condé Nast
  Publications: page 132
Chris Barker: cover, back cover and pages 2-3, 39, 41, 48,
  49, 57, 66-7, 94-113, 116, 125-29, 131, 162, 185, 189
Blue Sky Holidays Ltd: page 53
Barry Bullough: cover, back cover and pages 2, 6, 7, 9,
  10, 11, 13, 15, 16, 21, 25, 28, 176, 178, 180-81
Cedar Falls Health Club: pages 144, 155, 188
Clarins Ltd: page 151
Creasy Public Relations: page 55
Elizabeth Arden: pages 142, 143
Evian: page 114
Joshua and David Galvin: pages 157, 161
Brian Gibbs: pages 50, 51, 65, 85
Hawaiian Tropic: page 82
The Image Bank: pages 134, 145
Le coq sportif: pages 2, 72, 73
Tony McGee: pages 3, 66, 88-93
L'Oréal: pages 45, 135, 157, 160, 161
Raleigh: page 54
Rex Features: page 36
Al Rockall: back cover and pages 3, 35, 190, 191
Mark Shearman: pages 63, 79, 87, 164, 182, 186
Slazengers Ltd: page 47
Trevor Strutton: page 47
Vision International: pages 30, 38, 60, 61, 75, 77, 80, 81,
  83, 164, 185

Work-out and cover model: Cheryl Holmes
Yoga model: Barbara Gurawska
Weights model: Vikki Galbraith
Make-up artist: Christina Saunders
Beauty model: Caroline Williams

Tables on pages 17, 23 and 33 are reproduced from the
Manual of Nutrition by permission of the Controller of
Her Majesty's Stationery Office.

Work-out and weight-training sequences were performed
at Holmes Place Health Club, London SW10

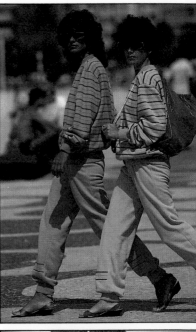

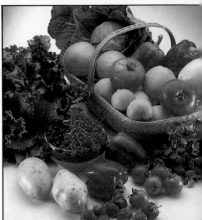

First published in 1984
by William Collins Sons & Co Ltd
London · Glasgow · Sydney
Auckland · Johannesburg

© Sackville Design Group Ltd 1984

Designed and produced by Sackville Design Group Ltd
32-34 Great Titchfield Street, London W1P 7AD
Typeset in Zapf International by Sackville Design Group Ltd

Art director: Al Rockall
Illustrations: Al Rockall and Phil Evans
Editorial consultant: Jennifer Mulherin

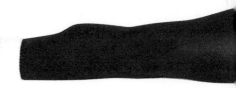

ISBN hb 0 00 411794 8
ISBN pb 0 00 411777 8

Printed in Great Britain by William Collins Sons & Co Ltd

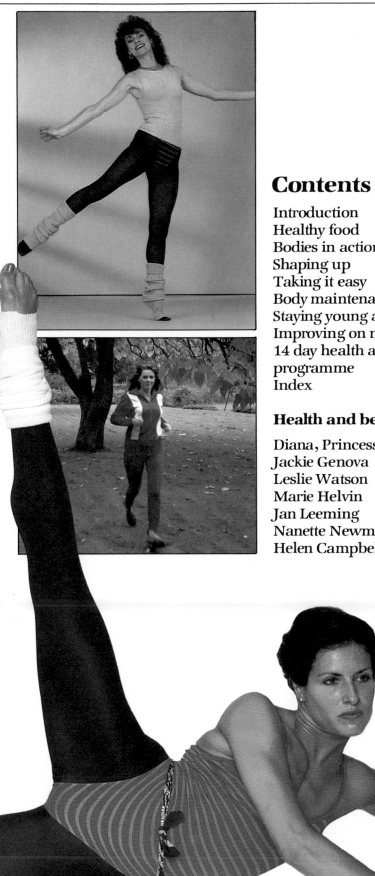

Contents

Health and beauty profiles

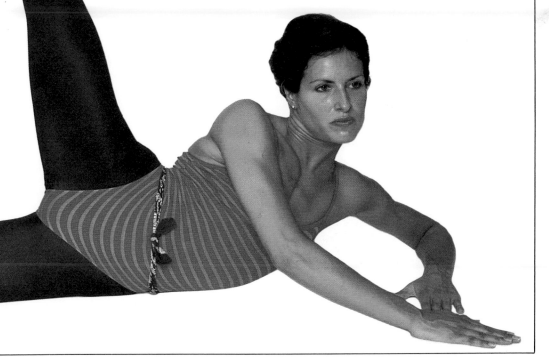

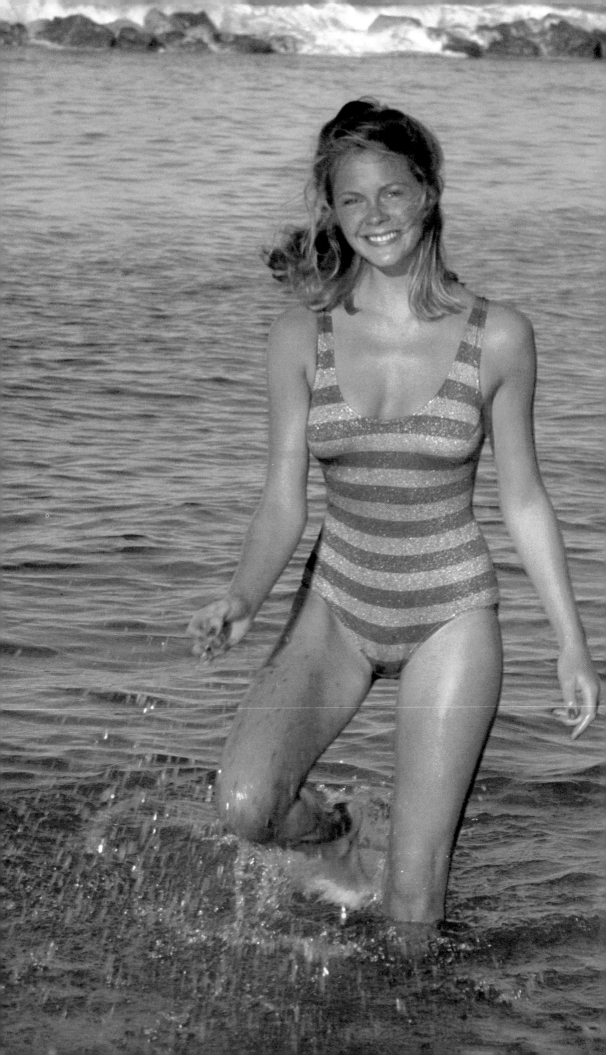

INTRODUCTION

Shape up to a new you

This book tells you how to get fit and healthy and how to look good. Real fitness and beauty come from within yourself — from a harmonious blending of body and mind, which makes you feel more confident and self-assured. When you are physically and mentally fit and active, you can come alive and feel and look radiant with health and the knowledge of your inner self. For this is a journey of self-discovery as you change your lifestyle and exchange your old unhealthy, sedentary habits for a new exciting way of life. You must learn how to enjoy sport and exercise, eat the natural, healthy way, relax and escape from stress, and look after your body and your health.

There are no set rules about how to go about this and you must choose your own personal route to health and fitness, but you will find plenty of advice and information from reading through the book and following the special 14-day health and beauty programme. Whatever your age, your shape, your level of activity or your lifestyle, you are potentially a fit, healthy and beautiful person — you *can* do it.

The philosophy outlined in the coming pages advocates a more natural, healthy way of life than most of us live. Our environment and personal lifestyle is of paramount importance to our level of fitness, health and beauty, but many women are plagued by anxieties, stress, fatigue and negativity — all endemic of modern urban living and a sedentary lifestyle. Our bodies and our moods are affected by the air we breathe, the food we eat, the stress to which we subject ourselves, and our lack of activity. The toxic fumes we inhale from the atmosphere and the chemicals in our diet can gradually poison our systems as pollutant waste products build up within our bodies and eventually affect our physical and mental health. Even the translucence and smoothness of your skin, the condition of your hair and the firmness of your body are influenced by environmental factors and our highly technological age.

Although we may feel powerless to prevent our air and food becoming contaminated, we can combat the damaging effects to some extent by improving our general level of physical fitness, eating a healthy wholefoods diet free from additives and chemicals, and practising body maintenance and preventive medicine in order to stay in good shape and to activate some amazing physiological changes within us that only healthy living can bring about. As you get slimmer, healthier and stronger, you will find that you have more drive and energy, even greater powers of concentration and increased self-esteem.

Feeling fit and looking good can change your life in other ways too — broadening your interests and experience, enabling you to meet new friends, altering your expectations, and bringing relief from stress and tension. You will also be better equipped to cope with the natural ageing process within your body and can help slow it down, as it is accelerated by poor health and a low level of physical fitness. Taking your health into your own hands and developing a new healthy lifestyle and beauty routine will change your life for the better, making it more enjoyable and rewarding.

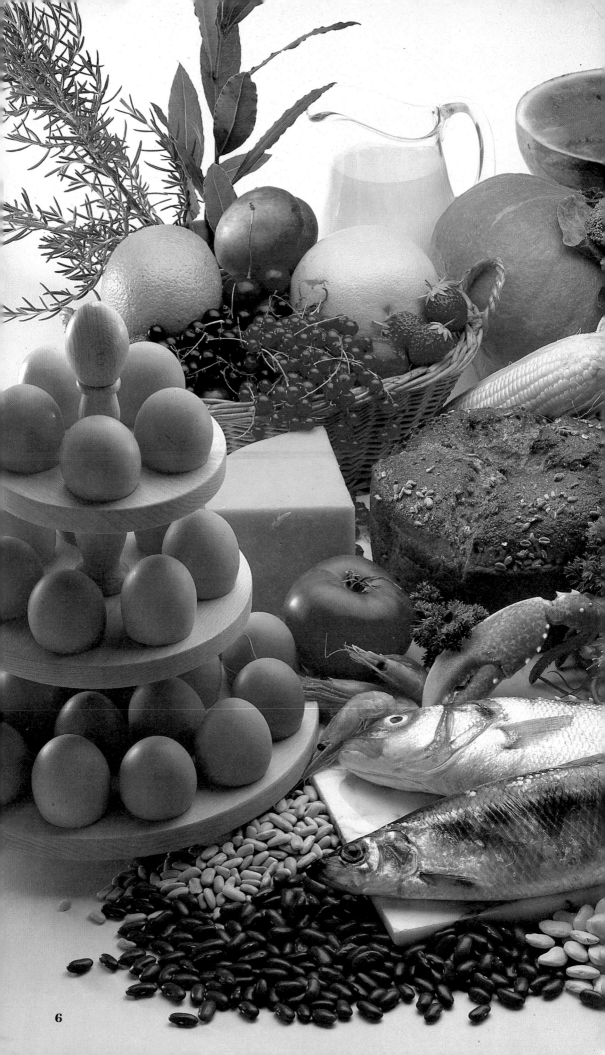

HEALTHY FOOD

A well balanced diet with all the essential nutrients our bodies need plays an important part in maintaining health, vitality and fitness. We need good food to fuel our bodies, to provide us with energy and to supply the building materials for growth and the healing properties for repair of tissues, bones, skin, muscles, hair and teeth. But although food is so essential for maintaining basic life processes and promoting health, it is surprising how little most people know about nutrition and its functions. We all know what we enjoy eating but how many of us understand the effects of our favourite foods on our bodies? What happens when we eat a hamburger and French fries, or a crisp green salad, for instance? To be really fit and healthy, you must understand the basic principles behind the food you eat and learn a little nutrition.

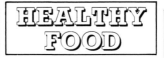

The essential nutrients we need for health and energy are proteins, carbohydrates, fats, vitamins, minerals and water. We can obtain all these from the food we eat, and a well-balanced diet should include adequate amounts of each. Within the body, each nutrient has a specific function and interacts with enzymes and digestive juices during the digestive process, is then broken down (for example, carbohydrates are turned into sugars, proteins into amino acids, and fats into fatty acids) and passed into the blood stream to be transported around the body to the cells and the liver.

Most people's diets are lacking in at least one nutrient, and vitamin and mineral deficiencies are common and contribute to many minor medical disorders, fatigue and depression. Most of us have a tendency to eat too much of the wrong foods and too little of the right ones. Most doctors now agree that the average diet is too high in fats, sugar and protein and too low in fibre foods, such as whole grains, fresh fruit and vegetables and dried legumes. Fats and sugar account for 64 per cent of the total calories consumed in the typical Western diet. This is obviously an unhealthy trend when we consider that the healthiest diets are high in fibre, vitamins and minerals, and low in fats, sugar and protein.

With 40 per cent of the adult population in Western countries overweight, obesity has become a major health problem and it can be seen that although we often over-eat many of us are under-nourished and we need to change our eating habits for our health's sake. Let's start by looking at the nutrients we obtain from food and how they affect our bodies.

Protein accounts for about 17 per cent of the body, including muscle tissue, skin, hair and nails. It is essential for life — for growth, for repair and maintenance of cells and tissues, for healthy blood and firm muscle tone. All proteins are made up of chains of amino acids, and all but eight of the 22 amino acids can be manufactured by the body. You can obtain the missing eight from the foods you eat. High biological chains, found in animal products (fish, meat, eggs and dairy foods) and soya beans, resemble the chains in our own bodies, whereas low biological protein chains, found in some vegetables, whole grains, nuts and seeds and dried legumes, are incomplete and have to be combined in the diet to make up the eight essential amino acids.

If you eat combinations of vegetable proteins wisely, you will obtain these amino acids with the bonus of the fibre and vitamins that these unrefined carbohydrate foods provide and without the saturated fats present in meat and most animal produce. Further protein can be obtained from low-fat animal sources such as cottage, curd and ricotta cheeses, skimmed milk and white fish. Protein is not stored in the body in the tissues as are sugars and fats, so you need to eat it regularly on a daily basis. Too little protein will lead eventually to a breakdown of muscle, whereas too much cannot be used by our bodies and puts a great strain on the liver and kidneys in removing the by-products of protein metabolism from the system. So cut down on your protein intake and limit yourself to about 40g/ 1½oz daily.

Carbohydrates provide us with energy and are converted by the body into glucose and glycogen to fuel our muscles, brain and nervous system. Excess carbohydrates that the body cannot use are stored as fat. Carbohydrates come in many forms, as starch, sugar or cellulose, the indigestible fibrous parts of plants. Starch and sugars are the biggest sources of carbohydrates in most people's diets, and the most dangerous ones. Sugar, in particular, and many other refined carbohydrates are virtually empty calories, and because they are rapidly converted into glucose and absorbed into the bloodstream in quick bursts, excessive intake may lead to blood sugar disorders, diabetes and obesity.

However, unrefined carbohydrates (whole grains, fresh fruit and vegetables, seeds, nuts and beans and pulses) are metabolised into glucose more slowly and released in a lower, steadier stream into the blood, providing us with a more sustained long-term supply of energy. They are also high in fibre which helps to regulate our bowels and keeps us slim

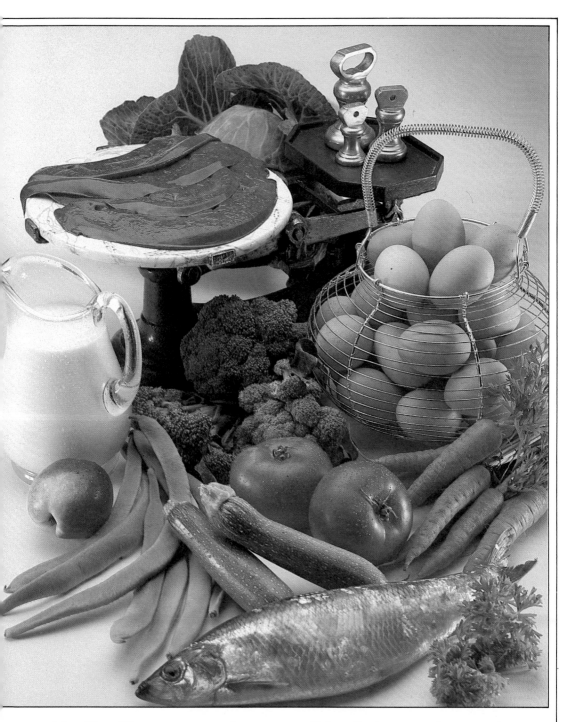

and healthy. There are suggestions on how to cut down on refined, processed foods and include more fibre in your diet on pages 20 and 18.

Fats are an important source of energy and also play a protective role in your body, helping to maintain vital organs, cell structure, nerves and body temperature and transporting the fat-soluble vitamins A, D, E and K. Fats are metabolised into glycerine and fatty acids during the digestive process for use by the body. However, excess fats are stored by the body as fat, and saturated fats can

All these foods are goood sources of vitamin A, which helps to protect your eyes and increases your resistance to infection and the effects of stress upon your body.

raise cholesterol levels in the blood, which may eventually lead to blocked arteries and atherosclerosis. Most people are now aware that although we need some fats for essential body maintenance and processes, excessive fats in our diet are detrimental to health and may play a significant part in heart disease, cancer and premature ageing.

Fats are available in three different forms: saturated, polyunsaturated and

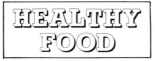
monounsaturated, and for more information on choosing and cooking with fats, you can refer to pages 19 and 23.

Vitamins are organic substances which you need to promote good health although they have no energy value. However, they do act as catalysts within the body and play an important role in the biochemical processes that release energy. Vitamins may be water-soluble or fat-soluble and are provided by the food we eat. The water-soluble B-complex, C and bio-flavonoid vitamins have to be taken daily in food as they are not stored by the body, whereas vitamins A, D, E and K, the fat-soluble vitamins, are stored in the fatty tissues. Our vitamin requirements vary according to our age, sex, level of activity and physical condition, but you should try to include foods containing the whole range of vitamins in your diet every day if you want to stay healthy, energetic and youthful. To help you choose the right foods, here is some more detailed information on the different vitamins and their role and functions.

Vitamin A is a colourless substance made from carotene, which is found in many orange, yellow and green vegetables and fruit, such as carrots, apricots, sweetcorn, cabbage and spinach. Carotene is broken down in the intestine and the liver to form vitamin A, which is important for maintaining clear skin, healthy hair, strong nails and good vision. You have probably heard the old saying about carrots helping us to see better in the dark — well, there is a great deal of truth in it as they are one of the best sources of vitamin A. This vitamin also helps protect us against stress, and builds up resistance to infection. Its deficiency can be detected in inflamed eyes, possibly with styes, dandruff, dry and flaky skin, loss of smell and general fatigue. To ensure a good supply of vitamin A, you should try to include some liver, milk, fish-liver oils, eggs, carrots, watercress, spinach, parsley, apricots and beans

Thiamine, or vitamin B1, is present in many whole grains and cereals as shown here. Liver, molasses, legumes and nuts are all good sources together with wholemeal bread.

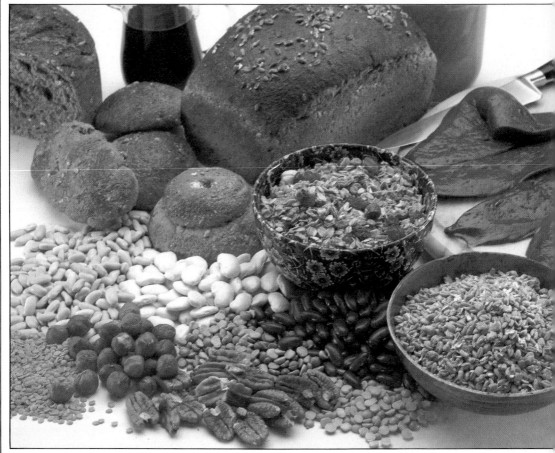

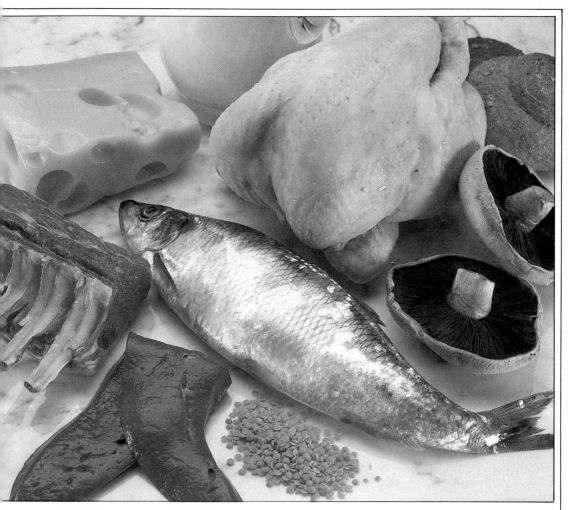

in your diet. You may find that you have a better supply of vitamin A in the summer when you tend to eat more fruit and salad stuffs, so try and consume more fresh vegetables and fruit, milk and liver in the winter to compensate for this. Lean muscle meat has little if any vitamin A although the livers from animals grazed in healthy organic pastures are a rich source.

B-complex vitamins, found in a wide range of foods, help perform many important functions in the body, especially burning carbohydrates, ensuring good metabolism and digestion, a healthy and efficient nervous system, clear skin, stamina, and maintenance of tissues, to name but a few.

Vitamin B1, or thiamine, is found in all seeds, nuts, grains, cereals and legumes as well as brewer's yeast, liver, kidneys, heart and pork, breakfast cereals and peanut butter. Some wholemeal bread, muesli and another thiamine-rich food will ensure that you satisfy your daily needs. If you are embarking on a fitness programme, it is particularly important

Most of us get adequate amounts of niacin, another B-complex vitamin, by eating a well-balanced diet of cheese, fish and meat.

to take thiamine as it helps you obtain maximum energy from your diet.

Vitamin B2, or riboflavin, occurs in liver, brewer's yeast, and most green vegetables. Milk is another good source but the vitamin can be destroyed by exposure to sunlight so never leave milk bottles out on the doorstep on a bright day. Bring them in quickly and store in a cold, dark place until use or, better still, buy cartons. Riboflavin helps in the metabolism of fats, proteins and carbohydrates and when it is deficient, these processes may be affected. It also plays an important role in beauty maintaining healthy skin and hair and preventing premature ageing.

Niacin, another B-complex vitamin, is found in liver, brewer's yeast, poultry, fish, lentils, milk, cheese and soya beans. Like riboflavin, it is essential to the breakdown of fats, proteins and carbohydrates and aids good skin. Lack

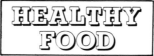

of niacin can cause digestive problems, skin disorders and general fatigue.

Vitamin B6 or pyridoxine, is important for growth in young children, as well as promoting good skin and guarding against depression and anaemia. Women taking the contraceptive pill are often advised to take supplements of this vitamin as well as folic acid, B12, zinc and vitamin C. Good sources of pyridoxine are liver, brewer's yeast, whole grains, most vegetables, muscle meats, fish, milk, bananas and nuts.

Vitamin B12, or cyanocobalamin, helps produce red blood cells and prevent pernicious anaemia, a condition in which imperfectly formed red blood cells are released into the bloodstream. It is also important for the metabolism of fats, proteins and carbohydrates and the synthesis of all new cells, together with folic acid, another B vitamin. Strict vegetarians and women taking the contraceptive pill are both likely to suffer from vitamin B12 and folic acid deficiency. Good sources of B12 are yeast, wheat germ, organ meats, milk, eggs, fish, meat and cheese.

Other B vitamins include pantothenic acid, biotin, choline and inositol, and these are found in a wide range of whole grains, dairy products, organ meats, vegetables and pulses. Together, they help in the process of staying healthy and fit and should be included in your diet on a daily basis as they are all water-soluble and any excess is eliminated by the body as waste. Many B vitamins are found in whole grains, usually in the outer layer and germ, which are not present in refined flour products, so always opt for whole grain bread, cakes, pasta and pastry made with 100 per cent wholemeal flour to ensure that you get an adequate supply of B vitamins.

Vitamin C, or ascorbic acid, has been hailed as a miraculous cure for many ills in recent years, including the common cold. But although it plays an important part in guarding against infection, healing wounds and fractures and maintaining healthy gums, its claim to be a cold cure is still not proven. It is especially helpful in keeping skin smooth and youthful-looking and maintaining collagen protein. The best sources of vitamin C are citrus fruits (oranges, grapefruits, lemons, limes and tangerines), blackcurrants, rosehips, strawberries, green vegetables, tomatoes and sprouted beans. It is water-soluble like the B vitamins and therefore some of the ascorbic acid may be lost during cooking, and vegetable water should be kept and used again as stock. Fruit that is left to ripen on the tree contains the most vitamin C, whereas many green vegetables contain more while they are still young and growing. Other factors affecting the vitamin content of foods include the use of fertilisers, the climate and the soil.

Vitamin D, the sunshine vitamin, is needed at all ages but particularly during infancy and childhood when young bones are growing. This is the anti-rickets vitamin as it plays a vital role in the absorption of calcium from food, and deficiencies can lead to bone malformation. Good sources are fish liver oils, milk, eggs and butter. A daily spoonful of cod or halibut liver oil, if you can bear it, will supply your needs, but another way of getting this vitamin is by interaction between the oils in your skin and sunlight.

Vitamin E, which is found in wheat germ, vegetable oils, whole grains and many green vegetables, is now a popular ingredient in many beauty and cosmetic preparations as it is thought to be an effective skin treatment and beauty aid which prevents polyunsaturated fats being oxidised in the body and helps keep skin young-looking and smooth. It helps protect us against air pollutants and is also useful to athletes and active poeple engaged in fitness programmes as it benefits the muscles' use of oxygen. So if you run regularly it is a good idea to take vitamin E, either as a supplement or, better still, as a spoonful of wheat germ sprinkled over muesli or yoghurt. There are also some excellent toasted wheat germ and honey breakfast cereals now available from many health food stores.

Vitamin K, together with calcium, is needed for normal blood clotting. It is present in yoghurt and kefir which has

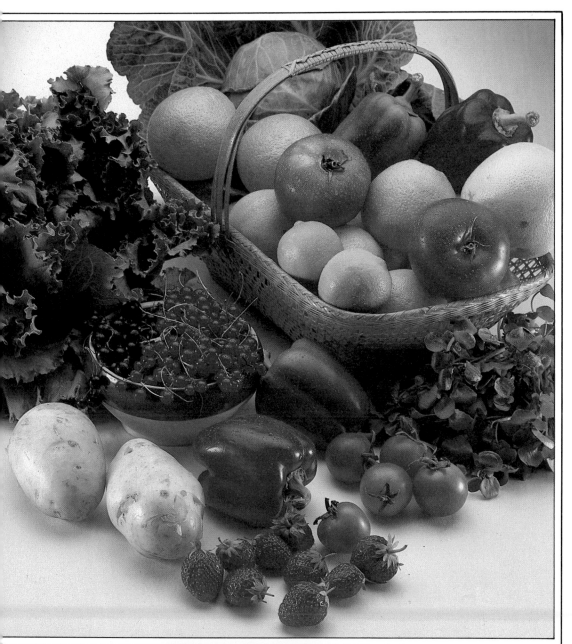

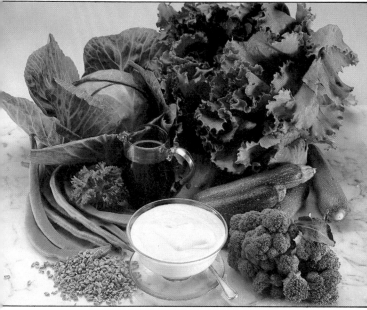

The basket of fresh fruit and vegetables (above) is rich in vitamin C, which helps guard against infection and keeps skin smooth and young-looking. Vitamin K (left) has an important role to play in blood clotting. Live yoghurt and green vegetables are the best sources of all.

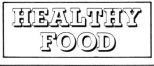
given rise to its reputation for promoting health and longevity. It is also found in liver, green vegetables, whole grain cereals and blackstrap molasses

Vitamin supplements

The shelves of health food stores and chemists are stacked with bottles of multi-coloured vitamin pills and supplements which many of us are persuaded to buy for our health's sake. But are vitamin supplements necessary and can they be dangerous in megadoses? It is generally agreed that most of us, if we eat a healthy, well-balanced diet, do not need vitamin supplementation. People who may benefit from extra vitamin intake include the elderly, pregnant and lactating women and those on the contraceptive pill who often have iron, folic acid and calcium deficiencies. Vitamins are needed by the body only in small quantities, and taking vitamins in excess of your requirements will have no nutritional benefits whatsoever. Fat-soluble ones may be stored in the body for future use while water-soluble ones will be eliminated in the usual way. Some vitamins, notably A and D, can even be toxic if taken in very large quantities. For example, scientific research with

Vitamin chart

Vitamins	Sources	Function	Deficiency	RDA
A	Fish liver oils, butter, milk, liver, egg yolks, cheese, yellow vegetables and fruits, dark green leafy vegetables	Normal eyesight, smooth skin, protection against infection	Poor night vision, sore eyes, fatigue, skin problems, poor teeth, dandruff	5,000iu
B1 Thiamine	Liver and organ meats, pork, wheat germ, whole grain cereals and bread molasses, nuts, seeds, soya beans and legumes, peanut butter	Healthy nervous system, stamina, aids digestion, good muscle tone	Beriberi, premature ageing, fatigue, muscular pain, loss of appetite and nausea	1.0mg
B2 Riboflavin	Meat, liver, organ meats, fish, eggs, milk, wheat germ, brewers yeast, leafy green vegetables	For many metabolic processes, tissue maintenance, Healthy skin, hair and nails	Eye infections, scaly skin, loss of hair, anaemia	1.5mg
Niacin	Meat, organ meats, liver poultry, fish, milk whole grain cereals and bread, peanuts, lentils, soya beans, brewers yeast, dark green vegetables	For metabolism of protein, fats, starch, improves circulation	Pellagra, skin and digestive problems, bad breath, fatigue	13mg
Pantothenic acid	Liver and organ meats, eggs, salmon, legumes, whole grain cereals, brewers yeast, peanuts	Anti-stress vitamin, good skin, healthy hair	Wrinkled skin, premature ageing, depression	5mg
B6 Pyridoxine	Meat, liver, organ meat, fish, brown rice, whole grain cereals, brewers yeast, soya beans, banana	For growth, synthesis of haemoglobin, formation of collagen	Anaemia, depression, bad skin, dandruff stretch marks	2.0mg
Folic acid	Liver, kidney, bran, brewers yeast, dark green leafy vegetables	For production of red blood cells	anaemia	400mcg
B12 Cyanocobalamin	Meat, liver, organ meats, egg yolks, sardines, tuna, salmon, wheat germ, brewers yeast, herring	For cell synthesis, red blood cell production	Pernicious anaemia fatigue, depression	3.0mcg
C (Ascorbic acid)	Citrus fruits, rose hips, blackcurrants, tomatoes, strawberries, raspberries green vegetables, potatoes, melon, peppers	Cementing cells, healthy teeth and gums, good skin. Anti stress vitamin	Scurvy	50mg
D	Fish liver oils, tuna, salmon, egg yolks, exposure to sunlight	For healthy bones and teeth and calcium absorption	Loss of calcium, rickets in children	400iu
E	Wheat germ, vegetable oils, whole grain cereals, nuts, eggs, legumes	Antioxidant in body	Wasting muscles, weak red blood cells	12iu
K	Yoghurt, eggs, green leafy vegetables, molasses, fish liver oils, alfalfa grass	For blood clotting, liver functioning	Excessive bleeding	200mcg

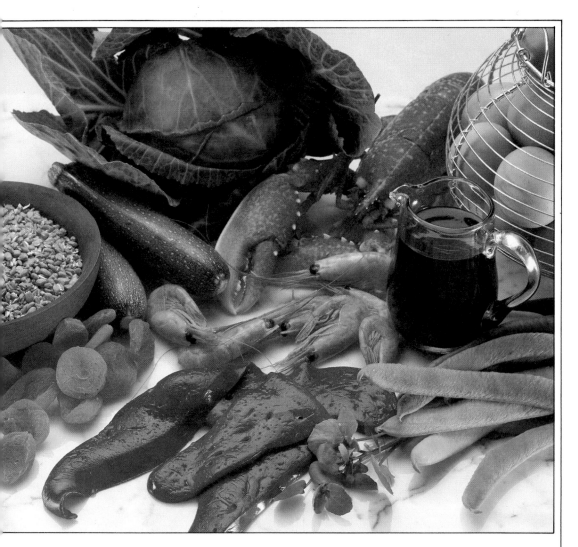

animals has shown that excessive vitamin A may be linked with birth defects.

It is often claimed that athletes and people who regularly engage in strenuous sport and exercise need vitamin supplementation for better performances, but most active, fit people are very health- and nutrition-conscious and probably satisfy all their vitamin requirements in their everyday diet. Of course, some athletes take vitamin pills religiously and swear by their beneficial effects but these may be psychologically rather than physically induced, and there is little scientific evidence to support their claims. Some people have been given a course of coloured water or even sugary pills under the impression that they are vitamin supplements and have improved their health or athletic performance as a result!

So before you buy your next batch of vitamin pills, ask yourself: 'Are they really necessary?' Or, better still, check with your doctor if you believe that you may have a deficiency to ensure that the correct pills in the right dosage are prescribed.

Iron is an important mineral for women, helping to protect them against anaemia. Above is a selection of common iron-rich foods which you should eat weekly.

Minerals are important nutrients for maintaining our general mental and physical well-being, yet they are only present in minute quantities in our bodies. They are extracted from the earth by plants and we, in turn, obtain them from the plant food we eat or from meat and dairy products from animals fed on plants. In the human body, they perform a wide range of functions — from keeping bones strong and healthy and regulating our metabolism, to affecting nerve transmission and the upkeep of cells, blood and muscles. As long as you eat a healthy balanced diet which is high in fresh unrefined foods, you will probably obtain all the minerals you need without resorting to supplements.

Calcium is vital for bone formation, strong teeth, good muscle tone and blood clotting. Most of the calcium in our bodies is

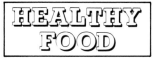
deposited in the bones and teeth (about 1.5kg/3lb), and scientific research suggests that children who eat calcium-rich food grow up to be tall. Calcium deficiencies can lead to bone deterioration, blood clotting, poor teeth and cramping of muscles. The best calcium foods, to eat are milk and cheeses, but yoghurt, nuts, whole grains, sprouted seeds, blackstrap molasses, clams, shrimps, sardines and other fish that can be eaten bones and all are also good sources. Powdered skimmed milk will provide you with daily calcium without the calories and fat of fresh milk. Your daily need of approximately 800mg will be provided by a healthy diet.

Chlorine is a gas found in vegetables such as celery, spinach, tomatoes and kelp. It combines with another element to form a chloride, as with sodium to form sodium chloride, or salt, another good source. It aids digestion and the regulation of our acid/alkali balance. We need only minute amounts, which are generally provided by salt in the diet.

Chromium helps in the regulation of blood sugar levels and in glucose uptake from the blood. It is only a trace element in spite of its important role in the body, and you should easily obtain all you need from eating either green vegetables, honey, blackstrap molasses, seafood, liver, brewer's yeast, whole grains, nuts or fruit.

Cobalt is important for affecting the functioning of vitamin B$_{12}$ in the body. Like chromium, it is only a trace element, and can be obtained from many green vegetables, whole grain cereals, fresh figs and some other fruits.

Copper is needed for the formation of red blood cells, for hair pigment and elastin in the skin. Good sources of copper include liver, shellfish, whole grain cereals, nuts, and brewer's yeast. We

It is unusual for anyone to lack sufficient phosphorus as it is found in most common foods, especially meat, fish, dairy foods and eggs, and has many important functions.

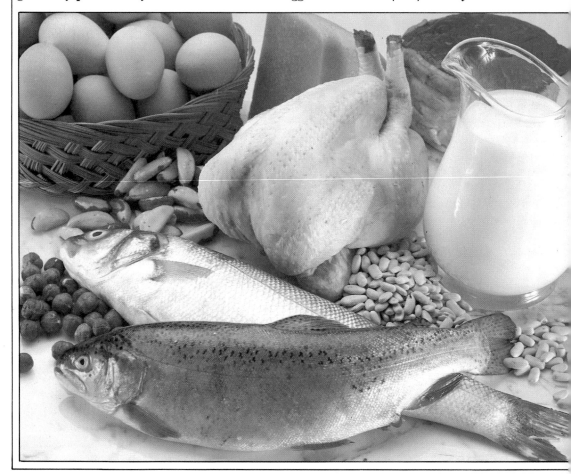

need only about 2mg per day but pregnant and menstruating women may require marginally more than this amount.

Fluorine is important for healthy teeth and gums and deificiencies may lead to tooth decay. However, as most drinking water is now fluorinated, it is unlikely that many people do not obtain sufficient fluoride. It is also present in shellfish and tea.

Iodine helps the thyroid gland to function efficiently and thus affects our growth and metabolism. The thyroid is the body's pacemaker and it may be under-active if you are lethargic, sleepy, out of condition and prone to put on weight easily. The best ways of obtaining iodine are by eating plenty of seafood, fresh fish, onions, fish liver oils and iodised salt as your body needs only a trace (about one-twentieth of a gram).

Iron is the anti-anaemia mineral and is especially important for women who lose blood every month during menstruation. In addition to its role in the formation of haemoglobin and carrying oxygen to the cells, it is also necessary for the metabolism of protein in the body and preventing general fatigue. Your body absorbs more iron from the food you eat when it is taken in conjunction with vitamin C. Iron-rich foods include liver, shellfish, egg yolks, blackstrap molasses, whole grains, dried apricots, green vegetables, sunflower seeds and potatoes. The recommended daily allowance is approximately 15-20mg.

Magnesium forms part of the green chlorophyll substance found in plants, and the best sources of this important mineral are green vegetables although it is also present in nuts, whole grains, molasses, bananas and many other fruits. It helps in the absorption and utilisation of other minerals, such as calcium and phosphorus, in building strong bones and in the functioning of muscles, nerves and the heart. Your daily need is about 30mg.

Manganese is important for activating enzymes, maintaining the reproductive system and for treating diabetes. Sources are whole grain cereals, leafy green vegetables, legumes, nuts and apricots. Only a trace is needed in your diet.

Foods	Sodium
Milk	50
Cheese, Cheddar	610
Eggs	137
Beef, average	53
Pork, average	63
Bacon	1,480
Chicken	70
Liver, average	84
Kidney, average	197
Haddock, fresh	120
Herring	67
Kipper	990
Butter, salted	870
Margarine	800
Potatoes	7
Brussels sprouts	4
Cauliflower	8
Peas, fresh	1
Peas, canned, processed	330
Mushrooms	9
Oranges	3
Peaches, canned	1
Prunes, dry	12
Cornflakes	1,160
Coffee, instant	41
Marmite	4,500
Milk chocolate	120

This table shows the sodium content in mg per 100g/4oz of some common foods. It may surprise you to learn its sources.

Phosphorus plays a whole array of important roles in the body, including maintaining the proper acid-alkali balance in the blood plasma, creating muscle energy, metabolising food, transporting substances through cell walls and keeping bones and teeth healthy. It is present in the nucleus of every cell in the body. We get all the phosphorus we need from milk, eggs, cheese, fish, whole grain cereals, nuts, legumes, liver, chicken and brewer's yeast, and deficiencies are rare.

Potassium, which is present in all living cells, helps balance sodium in the body and aids cell metabolism, muscle control and the production of energy. Deficiencies are unlikely as it is supplied by many foods, including muscle meats, fish, many fruits and vegetables, and whole grains.

Sodium plays a part in stabilising the body's acid/alkali balance, and in the maintenance of the muscles, nerves and blood. Excessive sodium can lead to fluid retention and aggravated high blood pressure — a good reason for cutting down on salt (sodium chloride). Sources are green vegetables, seafood, poultry, kelp and salt. Deficiencies may occur in hot climates owing to excessive perspiration.

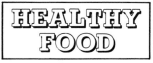

Sulphur aids in the formation of red blood cells and body tissues and the proper functioning of B-complex vitamins. It is thought to be good for the skin, hair and nails. Most of us receive all we need from eating a varied diet of eggs, fish, milk, meat, legumes and vegetables.

Zinc helps in the formation of enzymes, protein building, bone formation, detoxifying alcohol in the liver, transporting carbon dioxide and metabolising vitamin A. Women taking the contraceptive pill and those who are pregnant often need additional zinc, but the rest of us get enough of this important trace element from eating whole grain cereals, shellfish, nuts, seeds, meat and legumes.

Eating the right foods

As already shown, your level of health and fitness is dependent to some extent on eating the right foods — foods that are low in fat and high in fibre and natural goodness. This will soon become second nature to you as you begin to experience the benefits of your new way of eating and feel more vital and look better too. You may find that you sleep better, have more energy and feel slimmer, especially if you combine your new diet with increased exercise and sport. Here are some suggestions for you to follow to get you on the right road to health and fitness:

1 Eat more fibre

A healthy diet consists not only of getting the right nutrients but also eating foods which are high in fibre. This indigestible plant substance, or cellulose, provides us with roughage and helps us to stay slim, or even to lose weight in some cases. Fibre is not nourishing — its importance lies in its capacity to absorb liquid and become bulky as it passes through the intestinal tract. It speeds up the passage of waste products through the bowel and helps remove toxic matter. Whereas high-fibre foods make the journey through the body in less than 24 hours, low-fibre foods may take as long as three or four days and often result in constipation which has been linked with diverticular disease and cancer of the colon. Many doctors now believe that some of our so-called modern 'affluent diseases', such as diabetes, heart disease, hiatus hernia and obesity, are related to lack of dietary fibre. High-fibre foods are metabolised more slowly than refined carbohydrates and are thus a natural regulator in the system, releasing glucose for energy into the blood stream at a slower steadier rate.

Low-fibre foods are the result of modern food technology and they include most over-refined, high-calorie and convenience foods, such as sugar, cakes, biscuits and bread made with white refined flour, soft creamy desserts and many processed and canned products. High-fibre foods tend to be more chewy and filling and are thus an important slimming aid as they satisfy our appetites without filling us up with unwanted calories. Learn to recognise the fibre foods and include them in your diet. They include whole cereals such as whole wheat, brown rice, burghul, barley, oats and bran; most fresh fruit and vegetables; seeds and nuts; and dried beans and pulses. By eating wholemeal or granary bread every day made with 100 per cent stoneground wholemeal flour, including whole cereals (brown rice or baked potatoes in their jackets, for instance) in your main meal, eating fresh fruit for desserts and snacks, and a whole grain muesli-based breakfast cereal and plenty of fresh vegetables, you can ensure that your diet is high in fibre to keep you healthy and slim. Many modern reducing diets, such as the new F-plan one, are based on a high percentage of fibre in your diet and reforming your eating habits to maintain a slim figure.

2 Eat less protein

For years we have been told to include plenty of protein in our diet and as a result we have become a race of meat-eaters, but scientists have now proved that our need for protein has been grossly exaggerated and we eat far in excess of what our bodies require for health and maintenance. A recent report by the United Nations recommended a daily protein intake of only 36 grams, although most people eat four times this amount, and usually in the form of animal proteins which are high in saturated fats.

Research has shown that a high intake

of protein results in a negative mineral balance in the body as minerals are removed for the system and toxic by-products may accumulate from protein metabolism. Vegetable proteins, such as beans, pulses, whole grains, seeds and nuts, do not contain saturated fat and put less stress on the system, so try to eat some of these as well as animal proteins like meat, eggs and cheese. Reduce your meat-eating days per week and eat meat and fish in smaller amounts, filling up with plenty of fresh vegetables and cereals which are cheaper and more nourishing.

3 Eat less fat

The average Western diet is high in fat, so high, in fact, that it has been estimated that 40 per cent of our daily calorie intake in Britain, the United States and Australia comes from fat, and this is linked with the high incidence of obesity, heart disease, atherosclerosis and some forms of cancer which are prevalent in Western society but less common in countries with more 'primitive' diets. Too much saturated fat raises the blood cholesterol count and may eventually lead to blocked arteries or gall stones. Even if you cut out meat and dairy foods which are particularly high in saturated fats, and adopt a whole food regime of whole grain cereals, vegetables, nuts, seeds, fresh fruit, beans and pulses, your diet will still constitute between 10 and 20 per cent fats, so you do not need to eat a lot of additional fat to ensure that your body gets an adequate supply for nutrition and health.

Low-fat diets such as the Pritikin weight reducing plan are gaining in popularity although the controversy about the relative merits of saturated and polyunsaturated fats continues to rage. Basically, saturated fats are solid animal fats such as butter, hard margarine, cheese and cream. Poly-unsaturated fats from vegetable sources, including safflower, corn and soya oils and some soft vegetable margarines, actually lower blood cholesterol levels, but new research has shown that they may be linked to premature ageing and cell destruction although this has still to be proved beyond any doubt. Monounsaturated fats such as olive oil are neutral.

Fats lurk unnoticed in many of the foods we eat, such as ice-cream, chocolate, cakes, fried foods, eggs, pastry and many sauces, as well as in meat and dairy products, so you probably eat a great deal more fat than you realise in the course of an average day. You can cut down on fats by substituting low-fat cheese (cottage cheese, quark, ricotta and *fromage frais*) for hard and creamy full-fat cheese, by eating low-fat yoghurt and skimmed milk, and less meat. Most white fish are low in fat as are vegetables, fruit, beans and pulses, grains and cereals. Nuts and seeds contain unsaturated natural oils and should be eaten in smaller quantities.

Try not to cook with cream — use yoghurt instead. You can stabilise it to avoid curdling by blending it with a little cornflour before adding to a cooking sauce or dish. Use cream only for family treats and special occasions. Instead of spreading butter thickly on bread and toast, use only a scraping or substitute a soft vegetable margarine. Cook foods in the minimum of oil or butter and use a non-stick pan without fat whenever possible.

4 Cut out sugar

In addition to giving us energy, sugar also contributes to tooth decay, diabetes, obesity, heart disease and many other modern diseases, for sugar is full of empty calories, particularly the refined white varieties which contain no goodness or nutrients at all. Brown sugar contains marginally more minerals but is still detrimental to health in large amounts. In the West, we eat about 57kg/126lb sugar each per year. Like fats, sugar is another invisible ingredient in many foods, especially jams, cakes, puddings, biscuits, soft drinks, canned fruit, many commercial breakfast cereals and some processed foods. So cut out sugar now — get used to sugarless tea and coffee, even if you have to phase it out gradually by using an artificial sweetener such as saccharin, and substitute honey, molasses and malt for sugar in cooking. Instead of cooling down with soft sugary drinks, try substituting natural mineral water and freshly squeezed fruit juices. If you get hungry between meals, try nibbling at an apple or fresh fruit, some unsalted nuts or raisins, sticks of raw vegetables — anything but sugary biscuits and cakes. Lastly, be aware of manufacturers' synonyms for sugar which are printed on packets and cartons, such as glucose, dextrose and corn syrup — they are all other names for sugar. By cutting out

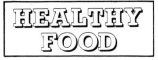

sugar, you will improve your health and your figure. You can obtain all the sugar your body needs for energy from fresh fruit and complex carbohydrates such as vegetables, grains and seeds, which are then converted into sugar by the body.

5 Eat less salt

Excessive salt can be a major factor in developing high blood pressure, which may lead in turn to heart disease and strokes. Salt and potassium are balanced within our diet and, if taken in excess, salt can damage this delicate equilibrium, sometimes causing fluid retention, kidney disorders and even muscle damage. By using less salt you can minimise these risks. It takes time to grow accustomed to unsalted foods so cut down gradually. Never leave the salt cellar on the table while you are eating — the food should be sufficiently salted during cooking without adding more at the table. Salt foods only lightly and start enjoying the real flavours of the ingredients and not just a salty taste. There are also vegetable-based substitutes which can be used for seasoning foods, available from many health food stores.

Make more use of herbs and spices, the natural seasonings, to enhance the flavour of food. Freshly ground spices and chopped fresh or dried herbs will add a delicious new dimension to your cooking. Most foods contain adequate amounts of sodium without the necessity of adding more salt. See the table on page 17.

6 Cut out processed foods

Most processed foods are high in salt, sugar and fats as well as chemical additives. Often lacking in fibre and natural goodness, processed foods have contributed significantly to the loss of quality and flavour of the food we eat and to the growth of many diseases, medical disorders and nutritional deficiencies. However, the most disturbing trend in food processing is the increasing use of additives of which there are over 3000 currently permissible in Britain alone. Although there are strict government regulations to control their use and they are all subject to rigorous testing, little is known about their long-term effects on the human body or how they interact with one another. They are usually included only in minute quantities in processed foods but they can build up in the body over a period of time and many are potentially toxic and may even be cancer-forming in certain instances. Read the labels and beware of sodium nitrite, found especially in processed cheeses and meats, BHT (a petroleum additive) and artificial food dyes and preservatives. All these preservatives, emulsifiers, flavourings, colourings, stabilisers and sweeteners which are supposed to enhance the appearance and flavour and extend the shelf-life of foods, might be harmful in the long run and are certainly less attractive and wholesome than fresh foods or natural ingredients. Stick to fresh fruit and vegetables, free-range eggs and poultry, freshly caught fish, soft cheeses that contain no additives, dried beans and pulses, sun-dried unsprayed dried fruits, cold-pressed vegetable oils, natural yoghurts, milk and unsalted butters. If you really do have to eat processed and convenience foods, do check that they contain no harmful additives or chemicals.

7 Drink less coffee and alcohol

Caffeine, found in coffee and to a lesser extent in tea and cocoa, and alcohol are both drugs which can cause damage to our bodies if taken in excess over a period of time. Both these psychoactive drugs are widely taken and socially acceptable but they do stimulate our nervous system, bringing about physiological changes in the body. Caffeine, for example, can speed up your heart beat, dispel feelings of tiredness and fatigue and may even relax muscles. However, it may also increase stomach acid, thus giving you a greater propensity to peptic ulcers. A great deal of research is still being carried out into the long-term effects of caffeine on the system, but any toxic drug which is taken regularly cannot be conducive to your health and physical well-being, so you would be well-advised to limit your coffee-drinking to one cup a day. As each cup contains about 150 milligrams of caffeine and a dose of 250 milligrams is considered high, this is within the safety limits. When you are thirsty or need a pep-up, try

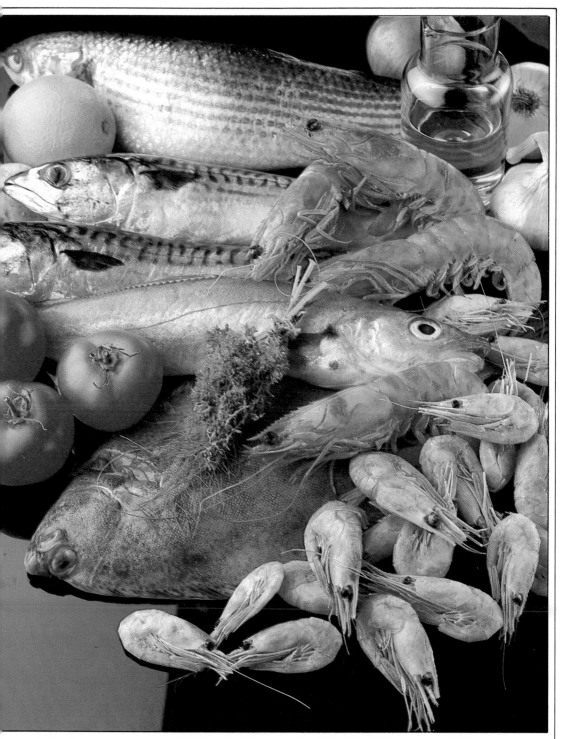

mineral water, fresh fruit and vegetable juices or herbal teas instead. There are also some good coffee substitutes available from many health food stores, which contain no caffeine

The effects of alcohol on the body are even more damaging and may be irreversible in the long-term. Many liver disorders are linked to a high and persistent intake of alcohol. Studies have shown that even social drinkers can sustain liver damage — you do not need to be an alcoholic. And your whole body is

Fish and shellfish are a healthy way of including protein in your diet and do not contain the saturated fat of red meat. In addition, they are a rich source of minerals, especially iodine and phosphorus.

affected if your liver suffers, with consequent hormonal imbalances, especially in women, and vitamin B deficiencies, fatigue and even depression. So try not to drink alcohol every day, or just enjoy one glass of wine or a beer with a meal. Lay

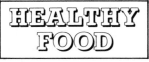

off spirits altogether, and at parties and social gatherings, stick to fruit juice or mineral water or one glass of white wine topped up with sparkling mineral water (spritzer) — they are all healthy, refreshing and are guaranteed not to give you an almighty headache the following morning!

8 Drink more mineral water

We often pride ourselves on the purity and fine quality of our drinking water and how much healthier it is than that in many Mediterranean, Latin American, Asian and African countries where boiling is an essential prerequisite to drinking. But did you know that our tap water contains many chemical pollutants (over 1500 are found in Britain alone) and these may gradually build up inside us over a long period of time? Sewage, industrial waste and toxic chemical materials all flow into the rivers and find their way eventually into our tap water. The chlorine with which it is treated to destroy any germs cannot counter chemical pollutants and may even react adversely with some of these toxic waste substances to produce more dangerous compounds, some of which are thought to be cancer-forming.

You can now buy water-softeners, but soft water may be correlated to a high incidence of heart attacks and strokes, as research has shown in some soft-water areas. It may contain tiny metal deposits from old-fashioned copper and lead piping and these can build up to hazardous health levels. If you suspect that the soft water in your area may be high in lead, then it is a good idea to have it tested by your local water authority. There are specific guidelines regarding lead concentration set down by the World Health Organisation. If in doubt, you can purchase a filter quite cheaply and fit it on to your taps.

Water is essential for good health — it accounts for two-thirds of our body weight, regulates our body temperature, helps in digestion, removing waste products from the tissues, lubricates joints and many other important processes. Therefore it is imperative that the water we drink should be pure and free from pollution. There is a wide range of bottled waters to choose from, including sparkling and still varieties. Many are rich in minerals and are obtainable from health food stores and most supermarkets. They come from natural springs in different countries, notably France where the ministry of public health tests all mineral water regularly and grades it according to its quality and purity. It may seem an extravagance at first, but at least you can be sure that the bottled water you buy is really healthy and pure unlike the polluted liquid out of your tap.

Remember also that not all of the water in our diet comes from the liquids we drink. Between 30 and 50 per cent of our daily water intake comes from food, and not just fruit and vegetables. Even an ordinary slice of bread is about 35 per cent water.

Guidelines for healthy eating

Here are some tips and useful advice on planning a healthy diet plus new ideas for delicious meals which can be quickly prepared with the minimum of fuss and effort. Cooking healthy meals need not be any more time-consuming than preparing so-called 'convenience foods' with their frightening array of chemical additives. Just follow the basic principles outlined above and use these practical tips to put them into operation.

1 Sweetening without sugar

Most of us have grown up with a sweet tooth and thus we find many unsweetened dishes unpalatable. Although we can eventually adapt to sugarless tea and coffee, it is harder to enjoy unsweetened cakes and desserts. Even if you are congratulating yourself on the fact that you eat only raw brown sugar with all its natural minerals and vitamins, it is still very concentrated and you would be better off without it for your health's sake. Honey is more nutritious and more readily digested by the body than are other sugars. It can be used as a substitute for sugar in most recipes, including cakes, puddings, cookies and stewed fruit. As a general rule, use half to three-quarters honey to the recommended weight of sugar. Honey can be mixed also with orange juice as a glaze for hams, or blended with fruit juice, soya sauce, garlic and herbs as a marinade for meat and poultry. Other natural sweeteners include malt extract and blackstrap molasses, concentrated fruit juices and dried fruits.

2 Cooking without fats

A set of good non-stick pans are a worthwhile investment for a healthy diet. Meat and poultry can be cooked in non-stick pans, or grilled, braised or baked either without fat or using only the minimum of a good polyunsaturated oil, such as sunflower or corn oils. Fish is particularly good grilled — you can stuff it with fresh herbs and a little lemon juice. A delicious alternative is to wrap up whole or filleted fish in foil parcels with chopped onion, herbs, mushrooms, lemon juice and white wine and bake for 15-20 minutes. Fish and meat can be cubed and threaded onto kebab skewers with fruit or vegetables and grilled until tender — serve with a crisp salad or plain boiled brown rice. You can also make many delicious, fatless hot meat and poultry stews and fruit *tagines* in the Middle Eastern manner by simply cooking slowly in water to bring out the real flavours of the ingredients. Buy a good cookery book on the subject

Oil-less salad dressings can be made with lemon juice and herbs; yoghurt and lemon juice; or puréed avocado with yoghurt. Eggs can be scrambled in a non-stick pan without butter, and vegetables can be steamed or boiled in the minimum of water until tender but crisp. Use skimmed milk instead of whole fresh milk in sauces, rice puddings, yoghurt-making, batters for crêpes, and hot drinks.

3 Preserving goodness and flavour

The natural goodness of many foods, particularly fruit and vegetables, can be destroyed or diminished by careless cooking and preparation. Always cut and prepare fruit and vegetables *immediately* before cooking or eating, as the vitamin content can be reduced considerably when they are cut and come into contact with the air. Cook vegetables in the minimum of water until *just* tender, and keep the vegetable cooking water for making stocks, sauces and gravies as it absorbs some of the vitamins. Steaming is an even more effective way of cooking vegetables and retaining their natural goodness. However, the best way to eat them is raw in salads, mixed with fruit, nuts, seeds and beans to make a nutritious meal.
Here are a few ideas for you to try out:
(1) Kidney beans, red and green pepper rings and parsley in a lemony dressing.
(2) Chicory, chopped apple, walnuts, sliced spring onions and chopped parsley in a yoghurt dressing.
(3) Cucumber, fresh dill, ground coriander and chopped green pepper in a yoghurt dressing.
(4) Wholemeal pasta shells or shapes, red pepper, spring onions, parsley and tuna fish chunks in a curry flavoured yoghurt dressing.
(5) Bean sprouts, orange segments, watercress, almonds and chopped onion in an orange and yoghurt dressing.
(6) Raw spinach leaves, sliced raw mushrooms, crisp crumbled bacon (grilled) in a lemony dressing.

This table shows recommended daily amounts of nutrients for women and men.

Age ranges years		Energy kcal	Protein g	Calcium mg	Iron mg	Vitamin A µg	Thiamine mg	Riboflavin mg	Vitamin C mg
Women									
18-54	Normal	2,150	54	500	12[2]	750	0.9	1.3	30
	Very active	2,500	62	500	12[2]	750	1.0	1.3	30
55-74		1,900	47	500	10	750	0.8	1.3	30
75 and over		1,680	42	500	10	750	0.7	1.3	30
Men									
18-34	Sedentary	2,510	62	500	10	750	1.0	1.6	30
	Very active	3,350	84	500	10	750	1.3	1.6	30
36-64	Sedentary	2,400	60	500	10	750	1.0	1.6	30
	Very active	3,350	84	500	10	750	1.3	1.6	30
65-74		2,400	60	500	10	750	1.0	1.6	30
75 and over		2,150	54	500	10	750	0.9	1.6	30

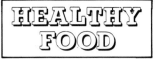

4 Cooking without meat

Cutting down on the amount of meat you eat is another way of reducing the fat in your diet and introducing more high-fibre, complex carbohydrate foods. Try to eat meatless meals at least three times a week and experiment with vegetables, brown rice and wholemeal pasta. Quiches and pies can be made with wholemeal pastry and filled with mushrooms, peppers, onions, spinach and sweetcorn in a cheese and egg custard. Aubergines, peppers, courgettes, tomatoes and cabbage are among the vegetables that can be stuffed with delicious fillings of onions, nuts, seeds, cheese, brown rice and dried fruit. Omelettes and savoury soufflés served with salad make light but sustaining meals. Beans and vegetables cooked in red wine make a tasty casserole, and wholemeal dough-based pizzas can be topped with unusual vegetables and cheese. Be brave and experiment with new ingredients and new ideas.

5 Healthy fast food

Fast food has become synonymous with 'junk food' in most people's minds, but cooking a delicious healthy meal can prove quicker than popping out to the local Macdonalds or reheating a frozen packaged convenience dish. Raw salads are quick and easy to prepare as are fresh fish baked *en papillote* (in foil), kebabs, barbecued grilled chicken, a brown rice risotto, wholemeal spaghetti tossed in tomato or mushroom sauce, or a vegetable gratin. And don't forget to make good use of your freezer — by cooking meals ahead when you have plenty of time and freezing them for when you are in a hurry, you can always ensure that you have some healthy food in the house and resist the temptation to succumb to convenience foods. Freezing does not affect significantly the nutritional value of most dishes and vegetables, so always keep some cooked vegetable quiches, wholemeal pizzas, bean casseroles and fruit pies in your freezer for emergencies.

Another useful labour-saving gadget is a food-processor which can take all the hard work out of chopping and grating fresh vegetables, puréeing soups, kneading wholemeal bread and whisking up vegetable dips and refreshing drinks. Some models even have a juice extractor attachment so that you can make your own fruit and vegetable juices.

6 Eating out

Unfortunately, many restaurants, apart from the vegetarian ones, are not very healthy eating-conscious, although the new trend towards *nouvelle cuisine* in many French restaurants has seen a move towards smaller portions and an emphasis on the freshness and natural qualities of the ingredients themselves. However, many dishes of meat, fish and poultry are still disguised in rich creamy sauces and desserts are still overwhelmingly high in fats and sugar. So what should you choose when you eat out? First course dishes of salads, fish and vegetable soups and consommés, shellfish, oysters, soufflés, melon, fruit cocktails, avocado and most vegetable dishes are obviously suitable. Grilled fish, shellfish, brochettes of meat or fish, liver and organ meats served with salad or vegetables all make good healthy main courses, while fresh fruit salad, or celery and a little cheese will round the meal off. It is really a matter of avoiding rich sauces and fried foods and puddings, and opting for plainer, simpler dishes.

Recipes

Here are some basic recipes for dishes to include in your weekly healthy diet. They are all easy to make — even the bread can be quickly mixed and kneaded in an electric food mixer or processor with a special dough blade attachment. You can make the muesli and granola breakfast cereals in bulk and store in airtight screwtop jars. They keep well for several weeks and can be served as breakfasts or desserts with skimmed milk or yoghurt, chopped fresh fruit, added bran and wheat germ.

Khoshaf, a dried fruit salad from the Middle East, and fresh fruit salad in fresh orange juice also make high-fibre, low-calorie desserts and you will soon prefer their naturally sweet fruity flavours to rich, cloying creamy puddings. Serve with plain fruit or home-made yoghurt.

Yoghurt is easy to make in a large thermos flask or a special yoghurt-maker.

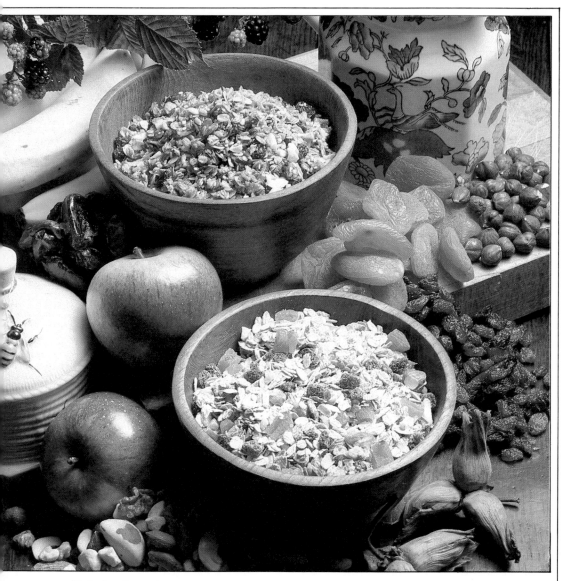

Keep a little back each time as a starter for your next batch. Flavour your home-made yoghurt with chopped fruit, honey, nuts, seeds and home-made muesli and granola. Serve it for breakfast, dessert or in smaller quantities as a snack between meals when you are starving!

Most seasonal salads can be served with a low-calorie yoghurt dressing, flavoured with lemon or lime juice or chopped fresh herbs, including mint, coriander, parsley, basil and tarragon. For really healthy salads, grow your own vegetables and eat them young, crisp and tender, or seek out the organically grown ones in your local health food store. If you buy supermarket and shop vegetables, always wash them thoroughly before using as they may have been sprayed with chemicals.

Home-made bread is always a treat, even when you make up a batch every week, and there is no more delicious aroma than that of warm fragrant loaves

Muesli and granola (background) are both healthy high-fibre ways to start the day. Add fresh fruit, milk, honey and yoghurt for extra goodness and flavour.

just out of the oven. By making your own bread, you can ensure that you use only the very best ingredients — 100 per cent wholemeal flour, added wheat germ, bran and cracked wheat (optional) and molasses, malt, herbs, spices, dried fruit, grated cheese, chopped nuts and seeds to enrich the flavour of the mixture. Bread need not be a chore if you plan it carefully. It takes about 10-15 minutes to mix and knead (five in a food processor). Leave it in a warm place to rise for an hour while you get on with other things, then knock it back (five minutes), leave to 'prove' (double in size again) for 30 minutes, and then bake for 30 minutes in a hot oven and, hey presto, you have lovely fresh loaves. Although it is a lengthy process, it

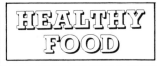

can be left on its own for most of the time and you are free to work, cook, shop, garden, clean or whatever. By doubling the mixture, you can make extra loaves and freeze what you don't want to eat straight away for future consumption. Home-made bread is very moist and keeps well (much better than commercially produced bread from a bakery) and it will be fresh and good enough to eat five days or more after baking.

Muesli

350g/12oz/4 cups jumbo oats
75g/3oz/$\frac{3}{4}$ cup rye flakes
50g/2oz/$\frac{2}{3}$ cup bran
25g/1oz/$\frac{1}{3}$ cup wheat germ
100g/4oz/$\frac{2}{3}$ cup raisins
100g/4oz/$\frac{2}{3}$ cup chopped dried dates
50g/2oz/$\frac{1}{2}$ cup chopped hazelnuts
50g/2oz/$\frac{1}{2}$ cup walnuts
25g/1oz/$\frac{1}{4}$ cup cashew nuts
50g/2oz/$\frac{1}{2}$ cup Brazil nuts
50g/2oz/$\frac{3}{8}$ cup chopped dried apricots

Mix all the ingredients together and store in a large airtight container. Serve as a breakfast cereal or as a dessert with milk, yoghurt and fruit. The muesli will stay fresh for about 4 weeks if stored correctly.

Makes approximately 1kg/2lb muesli

Granola

50g/2oz/$\frac{2}{3}$ cup bran
25g/1oz/$\frac{1}{3}$ cup wheat germ
50g/2oz/$\frac{1}{2}$ cup chopped hazelnuts
100g/4oz/$1\frac{1}{4}$ cups desiccated coconut
2.5ml/$\frac{1}{2}$ teaspoon salt
50g/2oz sesame seeds
100ml/4floz/$\frac{1}{2}$ cup vegetable oil
100ml/4floz/$\frac{1}{2}$ cup honey
2-3 drops vanilla essence
150g/5oz/$\frac{3}{4}$ cup raisins
50g/2oz/$\frac{1}{2}$ cup chopped Brazil nuts
30ml/2 tablespoons chopped cashew nuts

Mix the jumbo oats, bran, wheat germ, hazelnuts, coconut, salt and sesame seeds in a large bowl. Heat the oil and honey together in a small pan over low heat until thoroughly blended. Add the vanilla essence and pour over the granola mixture. Mix well so that all the nuts, grains and seeds are well coated.

Spread this mixture over a shallow baking tin and bake in a preheated oven at 140°C, 275°F, gas 1 for 35-40 minutes, stirring occasionally. Cool the granola, stir in the raisins, Brazil and cashew nuts and store in an airtight container.

Makes approximately 1kg/2lb granola

Granary bread

1.5kg/3lb/13$\frac{1}{2}$ cups wholewheat flour
15ml/1 tablespoon salt
50g/2oz/$\frac{1}{4}$ cup vegetable margarine
350g/12oz/2 cups cracked wheat
25g/1oz/$\frac{1}{3}$ cup wheat germ
50g/2oz/$\frac{2}{3}$ cup bran
45ml/3 tablespoons dark brown sugar
30ml/2 tablespoons molasses
900ml/1$\frac{1}{2}$ pints/3$\frac{1}{4}$ cups warm water
40g/1$\frac{1}{2}$oz fresh yeast (or 20g/$\frac{3}{4}$oz dried yeast)
beaten egg, milk or salt water to glaze
cracked wheat for decoration

Place the flour and salt in a large mixing bowl and rub in the margarine. Stir in the cracked wheat, wheat germ, bran and brown sugar. Blend the molasses and warm water and add 30ml/2 tablespoons of this mixture to the fresh yeast and stir until mixed. If you are using dried yeast, sprinkle it onto the molasses and water mixture and leave in a warm place until it bubbles up the sides of the dish.

Make a well in the centre of the flour and dried ingredients and pour in the yeast and the remaining liquid. Mix to form a smooth dough which leaves the sides of the bowl clean. Add more water if necessary as the dough must not be dry. Turn out onto a lightly floured board and knead well. Return the kneaded dough to the bowl, cover with a cloth and leave at room temperature for 2 hours. Alternatively, for a quick rise, place the bowl in a warm place and leave for about 45 minutes until well-risen.

Knock the dough back and knead again. Cut into 3 pieces and shape into loaves. Put each in a well-greased 450g/1lb loaf tin and leave to prove until the dough rises to the top of the tins. Glaze the tops with beaten egg, milk or salt water. Sprinkle over a little cracked wheat if wished for an attractive finish. Place in a preheated oven at 230°C, 450°F, gas 8 for

30-45 minutes. The loaves are cooked when they are brown and crusty on the outside and the base sounds hollow when tapped with your knuckles. Cool on a wire tray.

Makes three 450g/1lb loaves

Basic wholemeal bread

450g/1lb/4$\frac{1}{2}$ cups wholemeal flour
2.5ml/$\frac{1}{2}$ teaspoon salt
25g/1oz/2tablespoons margarine or lard/shortening
15g/$\frac{1}{2}$oz fresh yeast or
10ml/2 teaspoons dried yeast or
1 packet prepared fermipan yeast
2.5ml/$\frac{1}{2}$ teaspoon sugar
300ml/$\frac{1}{2}$ pint/1$\frac{1}{4}$ cups tepid water
milk or beaten egg to glaze

Tip the flour and salt into a mixing bowl and rub in the fat. Blend the fresh yeast with the sugar and tepid water, or sprinkle the dried yeast onto the water in which the sugar has been dissolved and leave until frothy. Mix the yeast mixture into the flour to form a ball of dough and knead until smooth and elastic. Replace the dough in an oiled bowl, cover and leave in a warm place to rise (about 1 hour).

Turn the risen dough out onto a lightly floured surface and knock back to its original size, kneading lightly for 2-3 minutes. Shape into a large loaf or small rolls and place in a greased loaf tin or on greased baking sheets. Leave in a warm place to prove, covered with a cloth or some greased polythene. When the loaf rises to the top of the tin, glaze it with milk or beaten egg and bake near the top of a preheated oven at 230°C, 450°F, gas 8. After 15 minutes, reduce the temperature to 200°C, 400°F gas 6 for a further 30 minutes until the bread is cooked and turns out of the tin easily and the base sounds hollow when tapped with your knuckles. Turn the loaf out onto a wire tray and cool. Bread rolls will require less cooking time — test them after 25 minutes.

Makes one 450g/1lb loaf

Home-made yoghurt

550ml/1 pint/2$\frac{1}{2}$ cups milk
30ml/2 tablespoons natural live yoghurt
15ml/1 tablespoon skimmed milk powder

Heat the milk until it comes to the boil. Remove from the heat and cool to 43°C, 112°F. It is important to have the milk at the right temperature as yoghurt bacteria are destroyed at temperatures over 48°C, 120°F and are inactive below 32°C, 90°F, so midway between the two is ideal for the incubation period. Use a sugar thermometer to measure the temperature or dip your little finger into the warm milk. When you can hold it there for a slow count of 10, it is ready to use. Blend the natural yoghurt with the skimmed milk power (this is to thicken the yoghurt) until smooth, and stir into the warm milk. Pour into a warmed wide-necked thermos flask. Seal and leave for a minimum of 6 hours. When the yoghurt has thickened to a good custard-like consistency, transfer it to a clean container and refrigerate for 24 hours before eating. Do not incubate the yoghurt for too long in the thermos flask or it will turn sour — flavour the yoghurt with fresh fruit, honey, chopped nuts or muesli and granola.

Makes 550ml/1 pint/2$\frac{1}{2}$ cups yoghurt

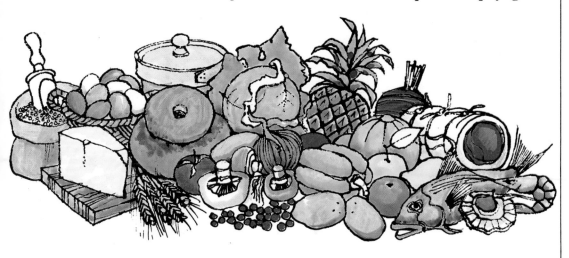

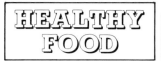
Yoghurt salad dressing

150ml/$\frac{1}{4}$ pint/$\frac{5}{8}$ cup natural yoghurt
salt and pepper
juice of $\frac{1}{2}$ small lemon
30ml/2 tablespoons chopped chives

Mix the yoghurt, seasoning, lemon juice and chives together and decorate with more chives if wished. You can add chopped spring onionss, crushed garlic or a pinch of mustard powder to vary the flavour. Serve with vegetable and bean salads.

Makes 150ml/$\frac{1}{4}$ pint/$\frac{5}{8}$ cup.

Fresh fruit salad

Various fresh fruits: bananas, sliced grapes, halved and pipped/seeded; apples, cored and cubed; pineapple chunks; oranges, peeled and segmented; kiwi fruit, peeled and sliced; melon, diced; pears, peeled, cored and cubed; peaches, sliced; apricots, stoned/pitted and quartered; cherries, stoned/pitted; strawberries; raspberries; mangoes and papayas, diced
Lemon juice to keep apple white
Honey to sweeten
Orange juice to pour over the salad

Prepare the fresh fruits and place in an attractive serving bowl. Sprinkle the fruits that discolour easily like bananas and apples with lemon juice to keep them white. Stir the honey into the orange juice and pour over the salad. This is more healthy and less sweet than making a traditional sugar syrup. Serve with plain or fruit yoghurt.

Khoshaf

450g/1lb/3 cups mixed dried fruits (apricots, prunes, figs, peaches, pears, raisins, apple rings)
50g/2oz/$\frac{1}{3}$ cup blanched almonds
45ml/3 tablespoons clear honey
grated rind and juice of $\frac{1}{2}$ lemon
2.5cm/1in cinnamon stick
15ml/1 tablespoon blossom water (optional)
25g/1oz/$\frac{1}{4}$ cup pistachio nuts

Cover the dried fruits with water and soak overnight. Place the fruit in its juice in an ovenproof dish with the almonds, honey, lemon rind and juice, cinnamon stick and blossom water (optional). Bring to the boil and then remove the pan from the heat, cover with a lid and place in a preheated oven at 170°C, 325°F, gas 3 for about 1 hour.

Add the pistachio nuts and cook for a further 30 minutes. Remove the cinnamon stick and serve the khoshaf hot or cold on its own or with thick yoghurt. The fruits should be very tender in their luminous golden syrup.

Serves 4

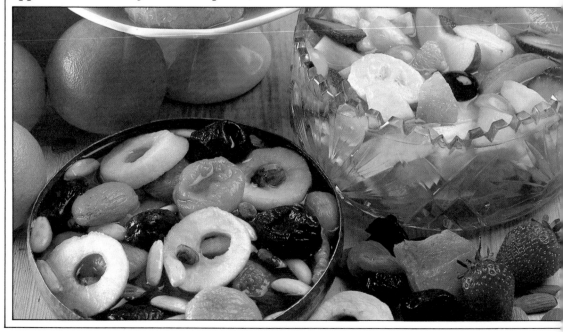

Slimming

A well-balanced healthy diet can help you to stay slim but what if you need to lose some weight first in your campaign to get fit and healthy? There are so many reducing diets to choose from — some sensible and others gimmicky — that you may have difficulty deciding on the right one. However, the best diet is the one that fits into your lifestyle and that you can comply with easily without making too many sacrifices. It should teach you good eating habits that you will keep long after the diet has finished and you have reached your target weight. In this way, you can stay slim and healthy, happy in the knowledge that you are eating the right foods and maintaining your new trim figure.

On-and-off dieting is not the best way to keep unwanted weight at bay — what you need is a diet to last a lifetime with new, enjoyable eating habits and good food. On the bookshelves and magazine acks you will see diets extolling the virtues of exotic fruits, cider vinegar, grapefruits and many other so-called magic ingredients that claim to really melt away fat; diets based on low fat, high and low protein, low carbohydrate and high fibre. Some are highly effective and others are just fads and gimmicks, so beware of eye-catching titles promising amazing weight losses in days and opt for tried and tested sensible, gradual reducing regimes which you feel sure that you can stick to.

In our society, slim is beautiful and most of us diet at least once a year in an effort to fit into last year's clothes or this year's holiday swimsuit. But slim is also healthy and you cannot feel as fit, active and vital as you would wish if you are carrying around excess unwanted weight. Obesity is fast becoming one the most common nutritional diseases of our time. While fat accounts for only about 15 per cent of the average person's body weight, it may be up to 50 per cent in the obese person and all this extra weight exerts an enormous strain on the system, making us easy prey for such diseases as diabetes, heart disease, and stroke. Bad diet and a sedentary existence are usually to blame. A diet high in sugar, fats, processed and refined foods combined with a desk job and a low level of activity inevitably leads to weight gain and a feeling of being unfit and out of condition.

Most diets are based on measuring calories and limit you to a fixed number of calories per day. A calorie is the amount of heat needed to raise the temperature of one gramme of water by 1°C, and is always measured in kilocalories (units of 1000 calories). Your body burns food to produce heat and energy, and if your calorie intake is greater than the number of calories your body burns, the excess is stored as fat. If, on the other hand, you take in fewer calories than your body needs, it has to draw on its fat reserves for energy and you lose weight. To understand about calories, you must learn to recognise and distinguish between the low and high calorie foods. All foods, with the exception of salt, contain calories, ranging from low-calorie foods such as lettuce, celery and mushrooms to high-calorie foods like butter and chocolate. Low-calorie foods can easily be turned into high-calorie meals by the cooking method you choose — whereas four raw mushrooms sliced up in a salad amount to only four calories, the same four mushrooms fried add up to a staggering total of 120 calories. Look at the calorie chart of basic foods to compare the calorie values of your favourite things and resolve to cut out the high-calorie items in favour of low-calorie fresh fruit and vegetables.

How much should you lose?

Your ideal weight is the one at which you feel normal and at your best, and which you can maintain long after your slimming diet has finished. You should not have to crash-diet every week for a couple of days to stay that way. Weight charts (see page 31) are useful as a general guide and it is easy to calculate the range into which your ideal weight should fall if you know your height and figure type — small, medium or large frame.

However, the best test is to stand naked in front of a full-length mirror and look at yourself critically. Ask yourself a few questions:
1   Do I need to lose weight all over?
2   Do I need to firm up saggy muscles?
3   How much weight do I need to lose?
Remember when you weigh yourself and set a target weight to aim for, that your weight fluctuates almost daily, depending on your menstrual cycle and the amount of fluid in your body. Fluid retention is a common problem for many women, and

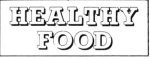
you may find that your weight drops dramatically in the first few days of your diet, but after the first week your weight loss is slower and more gradual. When we restrict our intake of food, we tend to lose water from our bodies first — body fat is burned up more slowly. When we eat too much salt, water accumulates in our bodies and we may swell up, particularly in the week preceding menstruation. This is not due to an excessive intake of water so continue drinking plenty of water as before — it will help detoxify your body and eliminate any waste — and cut down on salt instead. Restrict high-calorie drinks (soft drinks, alcohol, sugary tea and coffee) and choose mineral water instead. You need about 1.6 litres/3 pints a day for health — your body will get rid of the surplus. There is an old addage that drinking water washes away weight and scientists are now beginning to realise that there may be some truth in this.

When deciding your right weight, bear in mind that you may have problem areas where weight is concentrated, such as heavy thighs, a thick waistline, flabby upper arms or a droopy behind. Losing weight may be more difficult when it is not spread evenly across your body and you will have to combine your diet with special toning-up and firming exercises for these problem regions. Do not assume automatically that you know your height — we all shrink slightly as we get older and you may be shorter at forty than you were at twenty so measure it accurately before you weigh yourself and refer to the ideal weight charts. Remove your shoes and any heavy clothing before you get on the scales and make sure that they are properly adjusted and standing on a flat surface — all these factors can affect the reading. Stand tall on the scales and always weigh yourself at the same time of day. Weight can fluctuate in such a way that you weigh less in the morning before you eat than in the evening.

Most modern nutritionists and doctors agree that the most successful and healthy slimming diet is well-balanced in its nutrients, low in protein and fats and high in unrefined carbohydrates and fibre. It aims for steady, not dramatic, weight loss and enables you to change your eating habits gradually and to discover a new healthy way of eating. If such a diet is combined with an activity programme (keep-fit exercise, aerobics, California stretch work-out, jogging, cycling etc) you will quickly feel the benefits as you experience a new feeling of physical fitness, increased energy, vitality and emotional well-being. You will get a psychological boost from feeling slim and supple, and this new sense of achievement and well-being can permeate every aspect of your life — your motivations and ambitions, your attitude to work, your friendships and relationships with your family.

The same diet cannot work for everyone as we all have different personal tastes and eating patterns but there are certain basic rules that you should observe regardless of your own particular preferences and lifestyle.

1 Try to eat less at mealtimes and never accept second-helpings: select smaller portions and chew them slowly, really savouring every mouthful and concentrating on the flavours and textures of the foods. Always eat at the table, not with a

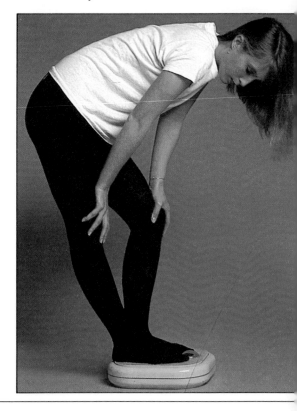

tray on your lap in front of the television, or in hastily snatched mouthfuls while working. If you do not concentrate on the food and you bolt it down, you are more likely to be unaware of what and how much you eat. Be conscious of what you eat and enjoy it — you will be less likely to over-eat and will feel more satisfied.

2 Try to eat three small meals a day rather than one big one: you are more prone to put on weight if you eat a whole day's calories at a single sitting. Smaller meals enable your metabolism to work in smaller spurts instead of having to do the job all at once. This is particularly true of people who skip lunch and have one large meal in the evening and then relax before going to bed — their bodies cannot burn up all the calories and some may be stored as fat. Also, never skip meals but get your stomach accustomed to regular, healthy eating.

3 Always eat a good breakfast: this will raise your blood sugar level and lift your energy. Research studies suggest that people who eat breakfast have more energy and better concentration at work than those who go without. There is no need to have a big fry-up full of calories — choose a bowl of high-fibre muesli with chopped fruit, milk or yoghurt, or a boiled egg and slice of wholemeal toast with orange juice. These are relatively low in calories and high in fibre and will satisfy any hunger pangs after several hours without food.

4 For snacks between meals, nibble at fresh fruit or raw vegetables rather than high-calorie sugary bisuits, chocolate bars, cakes and convenience foods. Fresh fruit will provide you with vitamins, minerals and roughage and take away any cravings — you will soon find that fruit is more refreshing and satisfying.

5 Instead of sweet, sugary and creamy desserts, opt for fresh fruit, either whole or cut up in orange juice to make a fresh fruit salad. Puddings account for many of the unwanted calories in our diet and should be regarded as treats for special occasions rather than everyday fare.

6 Eat more salads and vegetables: they are low in calories and quite filling as they require more chewing than soft, refined, foods. You can eat more food on a high-fibre slimming regime of 1000 calories a day than on a diet of 1000 calories based on refined foods. So you will feel less hungry as you lose weight.

7 Cut out soft drinks and alcohol for the duration of your diet and cut down on them afterwards also when you have achieved your ideal weight. They are full of empty calories and sugar with little or no nutritional goodness. Instead, drink mineral water and freshly squeezed fruit

Your ideal weight chart

Height		Small frame			Medium frame			Large frame		
1.45m	4ft 9in	42kg	6st	9lb	46.5kg	7st	5lb	50kg	7st	12lb
1.47m	4ft 10in	45.5kg	7st	2lb	48kg	7st	8lb	51.5kg	8st	1lb
1.50m	4ft 11in	47kg	7st	5lb	49.5kg	7st	11lb	52.5kg	8st	4lb
1.52m	5ft 0in	47.5kg	7st	7lb	51kg	8st	0lb	54kg	8st	7lb
1.55m	5ft 1in	49.5kg	7st	11lb	52.5kg	8st	3lb	55.5kg	8st	10lb
1.57m	5ft 2in	51kg	8st	0lb	54kg	8st	7lb	57kg	8st	13lb
1.60m	5ft 3in	52kg	8st	2lb	55kg	8st	9lb	58kg	9st	2lb
1.63m	5ft 4in	53kg	8st	5lb	56.5kg	8st	12lb	60kg	9st	6lb
1.65m	5ft 5in	54kg	8st	7lb	57.5kg	9st	1lb	62kg	9st	10lb
1.68m	5ft 6in	56.5kg	8st	12lb	61kg	9st	8lb	63.5kg	10st	0lb
1.70m	5ft 7in	57.5kg	9st	1lb	61.5kg	9st	9lb	65kg	10st	3lb
1.73m	5ft 8in	59kg	9st	4lb	62.5kg	9st	12lb	67kg	10st	7lb
1.75m	5ft 9in	61kg	9st	8lb	64.5kg	10st	2lb	68kg	10st	10lb
1.78m	5ft 10in	62.5kg	9st	11lb	66kg	10st	5lb	70.5kg	11st	1lb
1.80m	5ft 11in	64kg	10st	1lb	68kg	10st	10lb	72.5kg	11st	5lb
1.83m	6ft 0in	66kg	10st	5lb	70kg	11st	0lb	74kg	11st	9lb
1.85m	6ft 1in	67.5kg	10st	9lb	71kg	11st	2lb	76kg	11st	13lb
1.88m	6ft 2in	69.5kg	10st	13lb	74kg	11st	9lb	77.5kg	12st	3lb

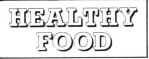

juices. Vegetable juices are also healthy and slimming and easy to make with a juice extractor.

8 Learn to read restaurant menus with a calorie-conscious eye: don't be tempted by French fries and rich sauces when low-calorie options are available. Opt for salad, shellfish and fruit starters; clear and fish soups; omelettes or grilled fish, meat or poultry for a main course; and fresh fruit salad or a *little* cheese and celery for dessert. If you don't want to appear the odd man out in a wine-drinking crowd, choose a spritzer — white wine topped up with sparkling mineral water — and keep topping it up with water, not more wine, throughout the meal. And never nibble at bread rolls, however tempting they may be.

9 Avoid the pitfalls of shopping: walk past tempting displays of attractive food on super- market shelves and buy *only* the items on your list. Don't be an impulse buyer. Better still, shop in an old-fashioned store where the goods are stocked out of reach behind the counter and the shopkeeper serves you — the tempatation to buy illicit food items is minimised. Shop after you have eaten to fight off temptation.

10 Keep active and busy: boredom is a common cause of over-eating. The busier you are, the less likelihood of raiding the refrigerator or the cookie-tin. As you step up your level of activity and spend more energy, you will probably find that your appetite diminishes and you want less, rather than more, food. Stress and tension may lead to compulsive eating also, so if you have a stressful job or are feeling particularly tense, get out and exercise — run, dance, work-out, cycle, swim, have a game of squash or tennis or just go for a good walk until you unwind and feel pleasantly invigorated and mentally refreshed. The power of exercise is amazing and sometimes you can literally feel the tensions and worries of the day slipping off you as you jog through the park or stretch in the gym. In fact, many psychiatrists, especially in the United States, are now advocating exercise and sport as a form of therapy for depression and stress. Also, don't start dieting if you are under great pressure or feeling depressed — you could add to your stress. Instead, wait until your problems are well under control.

Designing your own diet

If you wish to follow a rigid diet in which every mouthful of food you take throughout the day is stipulated and measured, then there are many books and diets from which to choose. However, most people find it hard to stick to a diet for precisely these reasons — because they have difficulty fitting it into their established working pattern or lifestyle. A certain amount of flexibility is important in any diet and it is no good expecting someone to cook a particular slimming lunch or arrange a special salad if he/she is out at work far from a kitchen. So it is sometimes a good idea to design your own diet and this is easily done with a little knowledge of calories and good nutrition.

We give you some suggestions below for your slimming diet which will enable you to lose weight gradually, say 2-3lb per week. It will help you to develop new healthier eating habits to stand you in good stead when you come off the diet and want to maintain your weight. If you want to lose only a few pounds and would prefer a crash diet, then there are plenty to choose from but this is a more sensible approach to weight reduction and healthy eating, and you can tailor it to suit your own personal food preferences and the pressures of everyday living.

Because it incorporates the principles of good nutrition and contains vitamins, minerals and fibre with a little protein and the minimum of fats and sugars, it will have beauty spin-offs as well, including improved, glowing skin, glossy hair and stronger nails. You may also find that you have more energy and vitality as you lose weight and discard the bad eating habits of the past.

Diet rules

1 You are allowed unlimited still (not sparkling) mineral water.
2 Snacks of fruit and raw vegetables are permissible between meals.
3 No tea, coffee (except decaffeinated) and soft drinks allowed.

Table showing composition per 28g/1oz of common foods	Energy kcal	Protein g	Fat g	Carbohydrate g	Calcium mg	Iron mg	Vitamin A µg	Thiamine mg	Riboflavin mg	Vitamin C mg
Milk										
Cream, double	127	0.4	13.7	0.6	14	0.1	142	0.01	0.02	0
Cream, single	55	0.7	5.5	0.9	22	0.1	44	0.01	0.03	0
Milk, liquid, whole	18	0.9	1.1	1.3	34	0	13[1]	0.01	0.05	0
Milk, dried, skimmed	101	10.3	0.4	15.0	337	0.1	0	0.12	0.45	2
Yoghurt, low-fat, natural	15	1.4	0.3	1.8	51	0	3	0.01	0.07	0
Yoghurt, low-fat, fruit,	27	1.4	0.3	5.1	45	0.1	6	0.01	0.07	1
Cheese										
Cheese, Cheddar	115	7.4	9.5	0	227	0.1	117	0.01	0.14	0
Cheese, cottage	27	3.8	1.1	0.4	17	0	12	0	0.05	0
Meat										
Beef, stewing steak, cooked	63	8.8	3.1	0	4	0.8	0	0.01	0.09	0
Chicken, roast, light meat	40	7.5	1.1	0	3	0.1	0	0.02	0.04	0
Kidney, average	26	4.6	0.8	0	2	1.7	34	0.11	0.54	3
Lamb, roast	83	6.5	6.3	0	2	0.6	0	0.02	0.07	0
Liver, fried	69	7.1	3.8	1.6	4	2.5	5,390	0.07	1.20	3
Fish										
White fish, filleted	21	4.9	0.2	0	5	0.1	0	0.02	0.02	0
Cod, fried in batter	56	5.6	2.9	2.1	23	0.1	0	0.01	0.03	0
Herring	66	4.8	5.2[5]	0	9	0.2	13	0	0.05	0
Eggs										
Eggs, fresh	42	3.5	3.1	0	15	0.6	40	0.02	0.13	0
Fats										
Butter	210	0.1	23.2	0	4	0	279	0	0	0
Lard; cooking fat; dripping	253	0	28.1	0	0	0	0	0	0	0
Margarine, average	207	0	23.0	0	1	0.1	255[3]	0	0	0
Oils, cooking and salad	255	0	28.3	0	0	0	0	0	0	0
Preserves										
Chocolate, milk	150	2.4	8.6	16.8	62	0.4	2	0.03	0.06	0
Honey	82	0.1	0	21.7	1	0.1	0	0	0.01	0
Sugar, white	112	0	0	29.8	1	0	0	0	0	0
Vegetables										
Beans, haricot, dry	77	6.1	0.4	12.9	51	1.9	0	0.13	0.04	0
Beans, runner	7	0.6	0	1.1	8	0.2	14	0.01	0.03	6
Beetroot, boiled	12	0.5	0	2.8	9	0.2	0	0	0.01	1
Brussels sprouts, boiled	5	0.8	0	0.5	7	0.2	19	0.02	0.03	10
Cabbage, green, boiled	5	0.5	0	0.7	11	0.1	14	0.01	0.01	6
Carrots, old	6	0.2	0	1.5	14	0.2	567	0.02	0.01	2
Cauliflower	4	0.5	0	0.4	6	0.1	1	0.03	0.03	18
Celery	3	0.3	0	0.4	15	0.2	0	0.01	0.01	2
Cucumber	2	0.1	0	0.4	5	0.1	0	0.01	0.01	2
Lentils, dry	86	6.8	0.3	15.1	11	2.2	3	0.14	0.06	0
Lettuce	3	0.3	0	0.3	6	0.3	47	0.02	0.02	4
Mushrooms	2	0.5	0	0	1	0.3	0	0.03	0.11	1
Onions	7	0.3	0	1.5	9	0.1	0	0.01	0.01	3
Peppers, green	3	0.3	0	0.6	2	0.1	9	0	0.01	28
Potatoes, boiled	22	0.4	0	5.6	1	0.1	0	0.02	0.01	1—5[8]
Potato chips, fried	72	1.1	3.1	10.6	4	0.2	0	0.03	0.01	2—6[8]
Spinach	6	0.8	0	0.8	20	0.9	284	0.03	0.06	17
Tomatoes	4	0.2	0	0.8	4	0.1	28	0.02	0.01	6
Watercress	4	0.8	0	0.2	62	0.5	142	0.03	0.03	17
Fruit										
Apples	13	0.1	0	3.4	1	0.1	1	0.01	0.01	1
Apricots, dried	52	1.4	0	12.3	26	1.2	170	0	0.06	0
Bananas	22	0.3	0	5.5	2	0.1	9	0.01	0.02	3
Blackcurrants	8	0.3	0	1.9	17	0.4	9	0.01	0.02	57
Dates, dried	70	0.6	0	18.1	19	0.5	3	0.02	0.01	0
Grapefruit	6	0.2	0	1.5	5	0.1	0	0.01	0.01	11
Lemon juice	2	0.1	0	0.5	2	0	0	0.1	0	14
Melon	6	0.2	0	1.5	5	0.1	50	0.01	0.01	7
Oranges	10	0.2	0	2.4	12	0.1	2	0.03	0.01	14
Orange juice, unsweetened	9	0.1	0	2.4	3	0.1	2	0.02	0.01	10
Peaches	10	0.2	0	2.6	1	0.1	24	0.01	0.01	2
Pears	12	0.1	0	3.0	2	0.1	1	0.01	0.01	1
Plums	9	0.2	0	2.2	3	0.1	10	0.01	0.01	1
Prunes, dried	46	0.7	0	11.4	11	0.8	45	0.03	0.06	0
Raspberries	7	0.03	0	1.6	12	0.3	4	0.01	0.01	0
Strawberries	8	0.2	0	1.8	6	0.2	1	0.01	0.01	17
Cereals										
Bread, white	66	2.2	0.5	14.1	28	0.5	0	0.05	0.01	0
Bread, wholemeal	61	2.5	0.8	11.8	6	0.7	0	0.07	0.02	0
Rice	102	1.8	0.3	24.6	1	0.1	0	0.02	0.01	0
Spaghetti	107	3.8	0.3	23.8	6	0.3	0	0.04	0.02	0
Beverages										
Coffee, ground, infusion	1	0.1	0	0.1	1	0	0	0	0.06	0
Coffee, instant powder	28	4.1	0	3.1	45	1.2	0	0	0.03	0
Tea, dry	0	0	0	0	0	0	0	0	0.30[10]	0
Squash, fruit, undiluted	34	0	0	9.1	5	0.1	0	0	0	0
Alcoholic drinks (fl oz)										
Beer, keg bitter	0	0.1	0	0.6	2	0	0	0	0.01	0
Spirits, 70° proof	63	0	0	0	0	0	0	0	0	0
Wine, red	19	0.1	0	0.1	2	0.2	0	0	0.10	0

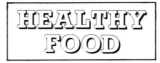
4 No alcohol.

5 Herbal teas, fruit and vegetable juices are permissible but no more than one only between meals.

6 No butter or low-fat spreads on bread and toast.

7 No frying in fats — grill, steam or cook in a non-stick pan or on a barbecue rack.

8 Use skimmed milk instead of whole fresh milk.

You may choose one from the following:

Breakfasts

1 A *little* unsweetened muesli, preferably home-made (about 40g/1½oz) mixed with wheat germ and bran and topped with natural yoghurt and 1 chopped fruit (eg. banana, apple, orange, peach) or strawberries, raspberries, blueberries. Mix with a little skimmed milk or orange juice (about 50ml/2floz).

2 1 boiled egg and 1 slice of wholemeal or granary bread spread with a scraping of honey.

3 1 poached egg on unbuttered wholemeal or granary toast.

4 1 small carton (150ml/¼ pint) natural yoghurt mixed with chopped fresh fruit, wheat germ, bran, 15ml/1 tablespoon sunflower/pumpkin/sesame seeds and topped with 5ml/1 teaspoon honey.

5 1 grapefruit half and 1 slice of wholemeal or granary bread spread with a mashed banana or a scraping of honey.

6 Stewed sun-dried prunes (and apricots if wished) in unsweetened liquid with 30ml/2 tablespoons yoghurt.

Drinks: either 1 small glass fruit juice or vegetable juice **or** 1 small cup herbal tea **or** juice of ½ lemon mixed with 1 glass warm water.

Lunches

1 Salad of raw vegetables: eg. sliced red and green pepper, fennel, cauliflower florets, zucchini, chicory, lettuce, spinach, Chinese leaves, watercress, mustard and cress, spring onions, celery, cucumber, sprouted seeds, tomatoes, raw mushrooms, shredded carrot, herbs, garlic yoghurt dressing (see page 28) or lemon juice + 1 slice wholemeal or granary bread and 1 fruit.

2 Raw vegetable salad with low-fat cottage or ricotta cheese and fruit

3 Omelette made with 2 small eggs and 5ml/1 teaspoon oil flavoured with sliced tomato and herbs.

4 Smoked salmon and raw vegetable salad.

5 Shrimps/prawns or lobster with raw vegetable salad.

6 Small can baked beans on wholemeal toast (most baked beans contain no artificial additives.

7 1 small potato baked in its skin topped with 15ml/1 tablespoon grated cheese **or** ricotta cheese and herbs with chopped tomato **or** chopped chives and natural yoghurt **and** raw vegetable salad.

8 275g/10oz any fresh fruit.

9 Small portion of tuna fish with raw vegetable salad.

10 One of the following liquidiser-chilled soups:
cucumber — blended with plain yoghurt, lemon juice, mint, garlic, coriander and black pepper
gazpacho — tomatoes blended with green pepper, spring onions, cucumber, lemon juice, herbs, black pepper and garlic

Drinks: either 1 small glass fruit vegetable juice **or** 1 small cup of herbal tea.

Packed lunches: most salads can be prepared in the morning before setting off for work and stored in an airtight plastic container. Prepare a dressing separately and place in a small screwtop jar and take to work with a fork.

Dinners

1 Grilled or poached white fish eg. sole, cod, haddock, turbot, monkfish, plaice flounder etc.

2 Grilled liver or kidney brochettes threaded onto skewers with onion quarters, tomatoes, peppers, mushrooms

3 Grilled white fish, shrimp or scallop kebabs threaded onto skewers with red and green peppers and onion quarters and brushed with lemon juice and fresh herbs.

4 Grilled chicken or turkey without skin **or** roasted in oven with herbs and lemon juice (no fat).

5 Poached or grilled scallops with lemon juice and herbs.
6 Omelette made with 2 small eggs and fresh herbs cooked in 5ml/1 teaspoon oil.
7 One green or red pepper filled with tomato, onions, mushrooms and herbs mixed with yoghurt and baked.
8 White fish fillet baked in foil with chopped onion, herbs and lemon juice.
9 Small salmon steak baked in foil with lemon juice and herbs.
10 Bean and vegetable casserole: mixed dried beans and vegetables baked in tomato sauce.

Plus: fresh raw vegetable salad **or** steamed crisp vegetables such as leeks, zucchini, French beans, mange-tout peas, garden peas, cauliflower, spinach, Brussels sprouts, celery, asparagus.
Plus: 1 slice wholemeal or granary bread **or** 1 small portion (50g/2oz) boiled brown rice.
Plus: 1 fruit

Drinks: either 1 small glass fruit or vegetable juice **or** 1 small cup herbal tea.

You can vary the dishes you choose from day to day and can stay on this diet for a month or more without suffering any ill-effects. On the contrary, you are likely to feel fitter and more healthy, especially if you start an exercise programme to supplement your diet. You need not feel as though you are starving because there is plenty of food—almost unlimited fresh fruit and salad vegatables, which are very filling as they are high in fibre and quite chewy. When you have reached your target weight, maintain that new slim figure by eating a healthy varied diet and cutting out fats, salt and processed foods as described previously. Staying slim and healthy is a new, more enjoyable way of eating, and although it is sometimes hard to break old habits and develop new ones it is well worth it for the increased health, youthfulness and energy that you will experience.

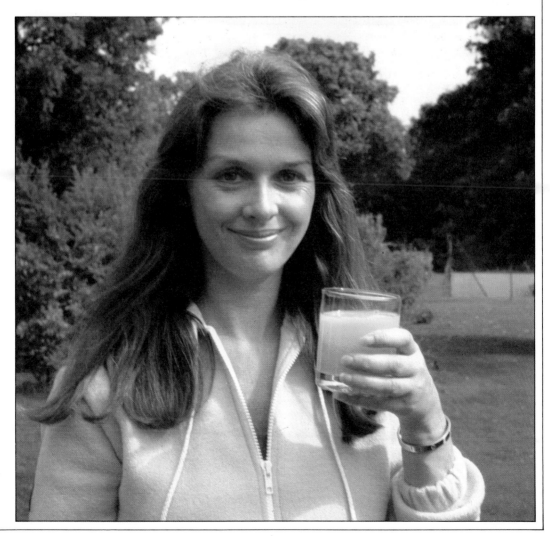

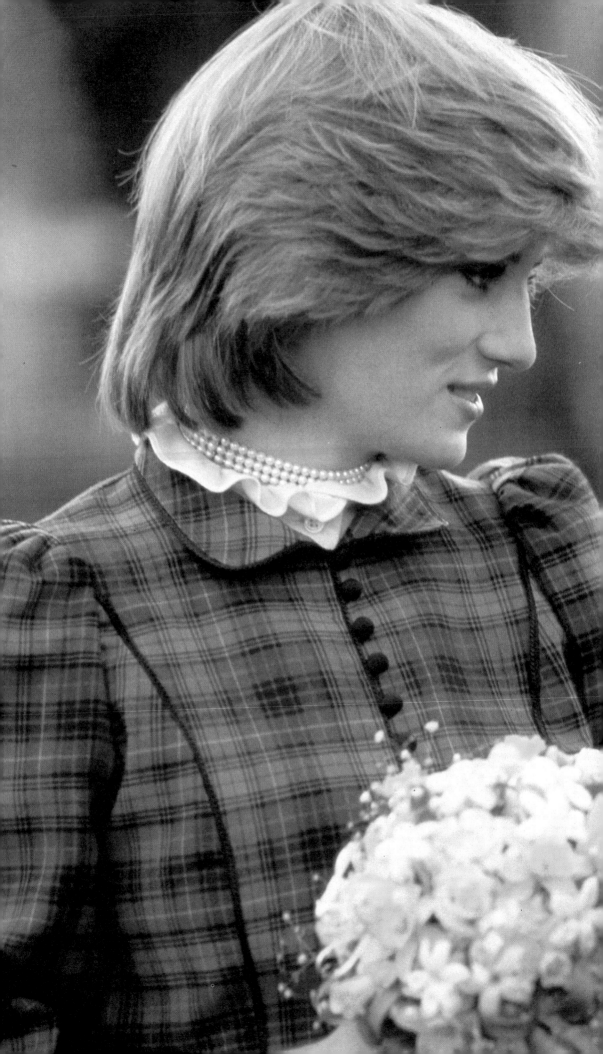

Diana, Princess of Wales

If you are what you eat, the Princess of Wales is a shining example to us all. She works hard at keeping her lovely looks and stunning figure by sticking to a simple eating routine, based on high protein foods such as fish and chicken, and by avoiding fatty foods.

Princess Diana admits to having a healthy appetite, and even confesses to the occasional yearning for tempting 'junk' food, in the form of hamburgers from certain famous fast food chains, but she shows great restraint in keeping these feelings in check! The words, 'I couldn't resist it' have ceased to be part of her vocabulary.

Before the Royal Wedding, Princess Diana successfully slimmed from 66kg/10st 5lb to 59kg/9st 4lb by keeping to a low fat diet of around 1,500 calories a day. Nowadays, her envied British size 10 figure is maintained by keeping her alcohol intake low — she usually opts for Malvern mineral water instead of wine at public functions — and by eating regular meals which include plenty of fresh vegetables and fruit. When she attends banquets, she is careful in her selection of courses. During their tour of Canada, the Prince and Princess attended a huge barbecue and, whilst others among the 1,500 distinguished guests tucked into enormous barbecued rib steaks — 1,500lbs of raw meat in all, cooked on a grill the length of a bus — the royal couple settled for more modest fare, choosing corn on the cob with a little Canadian salmon.

Breakfast for Princess Diana often consists of a high bran cereal, wholemeal bread and honey. One favourite food of hers is that famous high fibre product, the good old can of baked beans. Prince Charles was discovered buying a tin for her at a school fair, and told the children there, "The Princess loves them!"

Princess Diana's healthy attitude to life was emphasised when she left hospital only hours after the birth of her child, Prince William. The royal gynaecologist is keen on post-natal exercise and, within days, Diana was getting back into shape by working out the Jane Fonda way. Exercise forms a very important part in the lives of the health-conscious royals, and both the Prince and Princess of Wales enjoy the long-established royal habit of walking.

Princess Diana also loves to swim — probably the best all-round exercise one can do. When, as a child, she lived in Park House in Norfolk, the Royal Family were only a stone's throw away at Sandringham. Since there was no swimming pool at Sandringham, the Royal children were frequent visitors to the Park House pool. Nowadays, Diana still likes to swim daily, and aides preparing for royal tours make a point of checking out local facilities. Kensington Palace does not have a swimming pool, and so she uses the heated one at Buckingham Palace. When Diana was staying in Australia during the Commonwealth Tour, she was reported to have swum for 20 minutes nearly every day.

When she's in London, Princess Diana uses ballet and tap dancing to keep herself fit and in trim for gruelling tours and walkabouts, also firmly believing that dancing assists with correct breathing. On a visit to a ballet school, she told the pupils that she had wanted to be a ballet dancer herself once, but she had grown too tall to achieve her ambition! Her dancing, together with her diet and healthy attitude to life, pays excellent dividends, nevertheless. Her figure and her perfect complexion are the envy of many women throughout the world!

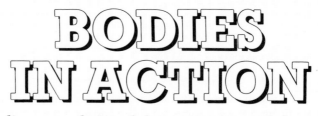

BODIES IN ACTION

Our bodies were designed for movement, and the more we move them the fitter, healthier, and stronger they become. Increasing numbers of people are discovering the joy and benefits of regular exercise as they take to the roads, swimming pools, tennis courts and work-out gyms in the pursuit of health and fitness. They know that physical fitness and the sense of well-being it promotes are the body's natural state and that most of us have become alienated from our physical selves. Exercise and movement reflect the physical side of our nature which, because most of us tend to lead sedentary lifestyles, is often neglected and under-valued in the modern world. However, a new consciousness is springing up and exercise is becoming a regular, indispensable part of many people's lives.

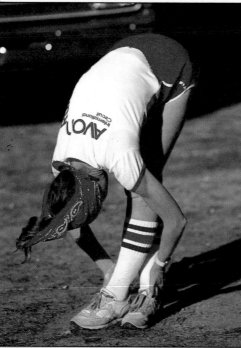

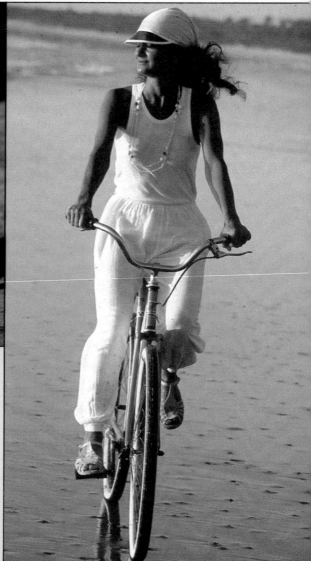

Aerobic exercise, such as cycling (right) or working-out in a gym (opposite) is a great way to keep in shape and develop cardiovascular fitness. It will make your body work efficiently and tone up sluggish muscles which are unused to physical activity. It is important to stretch out muscles (above) before you embark on any form of exercise in order to avoid stiffness and injury.

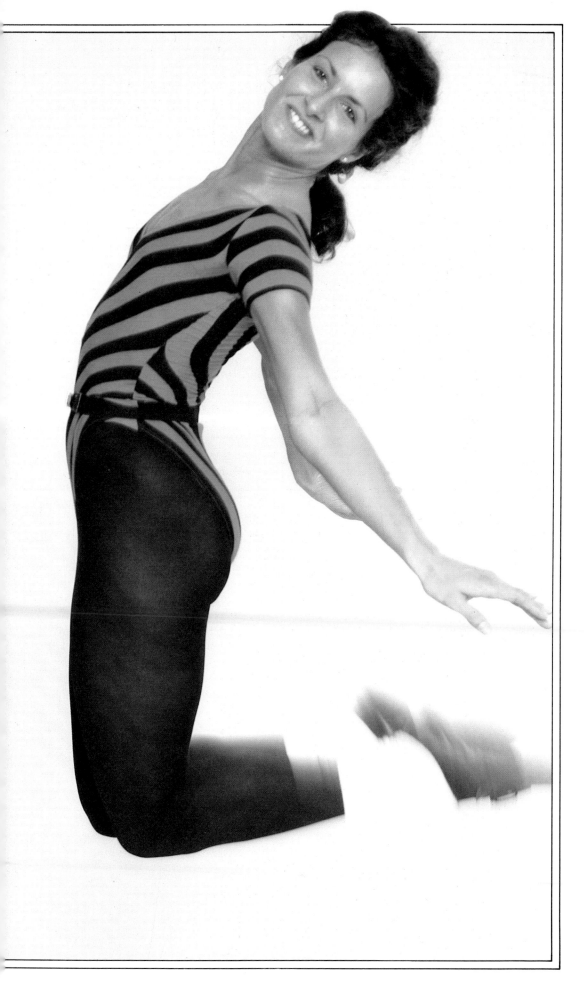

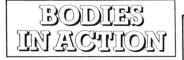

What are the reasons for this phenomenon? People are exercising to lose weight; to get physically healthy; to get into shape; to stay strong and youthful; to strengthen the heart and reduce the risk of developing heart disease and other modern degenerative illnesses; or because exercise is fun and fulfilling and they enjoy it. They come from all walks of life – professional people, doctors, lawyers, secretaries, teachers, housewives, students – and all ages, from young teenagers to men and women in their seventies and eighties, but they all share a common bond in their desire to get fit and healthy.

All doctors agree that physical activity is vital to our health. It can promote a strong heart and good circulation, a low resting heart rate, an increase in oxygen intake and efficiency in its processing by the body, firmer muscles, a more flexible and supple skeleton and a drop in blood pressure. It can also play an important part in delaying the ageing process and keeping bodies young and strong. Being fit also means feeling more vigorous and vital with increased stamina and energy for everything you tackle in your work and leisure hours. You may experience other spin-off effects of exercise too, such as a reduction in tension and stress as your propensity towards fatigue and depression decreases and your capacity for energy and enjoyment increases. Many people embarking on an exercise and fitness programme worry that they will feel tired and drained after hard physical activity, so they are pleasantly surprised when they learn that they have more energy, rather than less, for other things. Far from being worn out after a game of tennis, a work-out class or a 30 minutes' run, they feel fresh and invigorated. Even after a hard day at work, just 30 to 45 minutes of physical activity can make us feel refreshed and relaxed. Exercise is more effective than tranquillisers at promoting a sense of calm and well-being, and at making us more capable of dealing with the stresses and strains of everyday life. Problems and upsets assume less massive proportions, sleep comes easier and we feel less fatigued and irritable when we exercise regularly. Many people solve their work and home problems and worries as they jog around the roads or swim in their local pool, for exercise can affect our mood and our perceptions of ourselves, making us see things in a rosier light and encouraging us to be more positive and self-assured. Because we feel fitter, healthier and more confident, we experience enhanced mental energy and concentration. As we strive for and achieve new physical goals we can feel more confident about our mental and creative powers as well as our physical ones.

Primitive man was built for motion, and movement should be the most natural thing in the world for all of us, yet many people are so unfit that they even have difficulty climbing two or three flights of stairs yet alone engaging in some strenuous sport or exercise, such as running, swimming or cycling. The advent of the motor car and many labour- and energy-saving devices such as elevators, moving conveyer belt-type pavements and escalators, and the increase in sedentary office employment have led to a decrease in physical activity and fitness. How many of us drive to the shops or to work when they are within walking or cycling distance? How often do we elect to take the elevator instead of climbing the stairs, to stretch out in front of the TV on a fine day rather than go for a walk, or to telephone a neighbour for a chat when it is only a short walk away? But however inactive our jobs may be, it is important that we make the best use of our leisure time to get physically fit and stay healthy. In the past, most people had physically demanding jobs and occupations and their need for additional exercise was far less than it is today, when most people are eating more and are physically inactive. This trend has contributed to the increase in obesity and many health problems which are common in Western industrialised societies.

Physical inactivity leads to a reduction in body functions and decreased physical

An exercise bike at home or in the gym will help to keep you trim, and firm up leg and stomach muscles. Just 20 to 30 minutes' cycling a day three times a week will get you aerobically fit and develop strength.

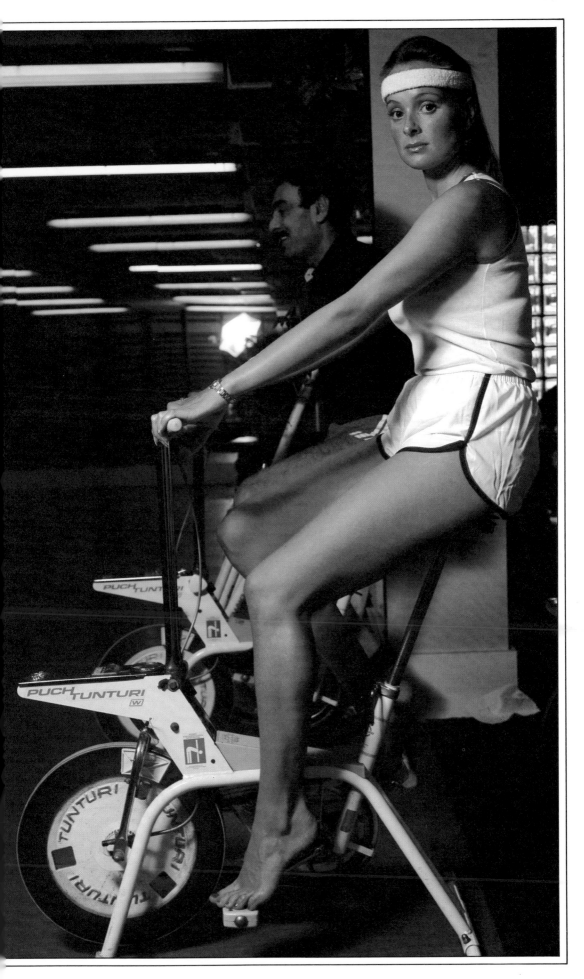

abilities as many inactive people soon realise when they start a regular exercise programme. Initially, their physical tolerance is low, they feel tired and breathless, their muscles feel stiff and sore and their bodies may ache. However, these symptoms do not persist and if they have the courage and determination to continue their exercise and physical training programme they will soon be rewarded by a greater capacity for hard physical work, increased energy and vitality and a firmer, trimmer body. The quality of their lives improves and they experience a new sense of mental and physical well-being. As a result of this momentous discovery, most make a lifelong commitment to exercise and it becomes more than just a regular swim or a run round the block but part of their overall philosophy for healthy and enjoyable living.

It has been claimed that you can get fit and strong in 30 minutes a week or less and there are countless books and magazine articles promising amazing physical transformations as inches drop away from your waistline and you get fitter and slimmer in a matter of weeks, if not days! But you only get out of exercise what you put into it, and you cannot expect to make progress and feel fitter and healthier if you play just one gentle game of badminton a week, say, or enjoy a round of golf at the weekend. To enjoy the benefits, you have to make exercise part of your weekly routine and do it regularly, at least three times a week. Start gradually, introducing physical activity slowly into your lifestyle, and build it up as you feel stronger and more supple. Embarking on a strenuous crash programme if you are very inactive can be painful and dangerous and you are likely to get injured or give up and return to your old sedentary lifestyle. Don't expect to feel marvellous straight away – your muscles will be unused to physical exertion and they will probably feel tight and sore at first and you may feel stiff the following day. The maxim to follow is 'train, don't strain'. Take it easily, building up gradually and within a few weeks your body will respond and you will feel more supple, energetic, and slimmer too.

The cumulative effects of exercise will

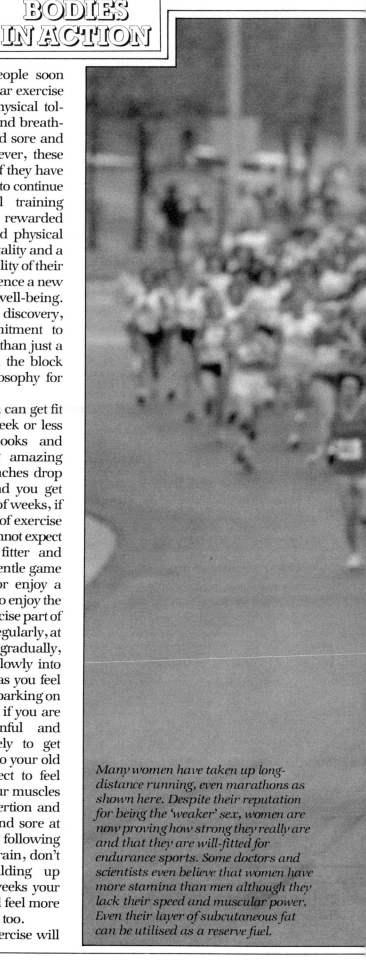

Many women have taken up long-distance running, even marathons as shown here. Despite their reputation for being the 'weaker' sex, women are now proving how strong they really are and that they are will-fitted for endurance sports. Some doctors and scientists even believe that women have more stamina than men although they lack their speed and muscular power. Even their layer of subcutaneous fat can be utilised as a reserve fuel.

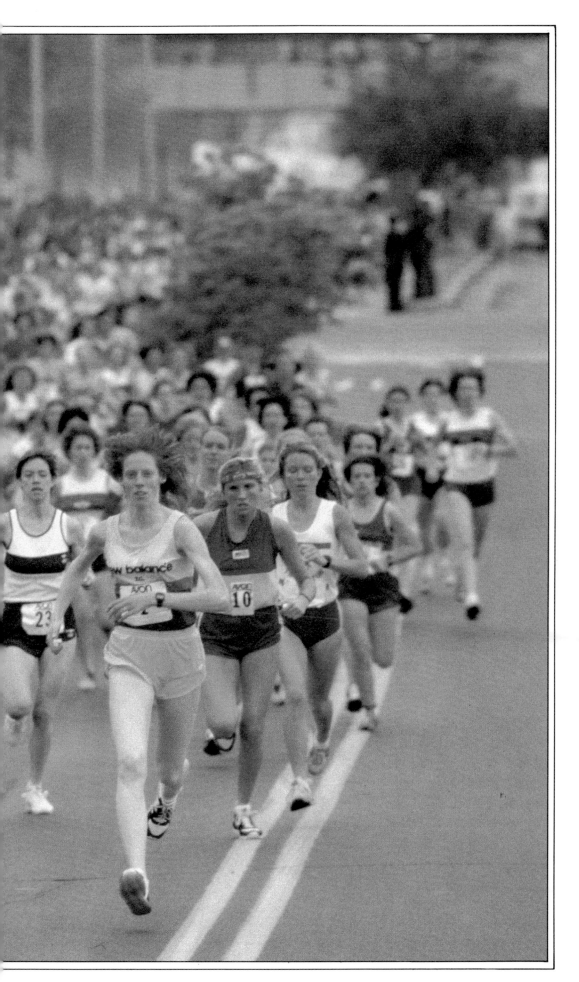

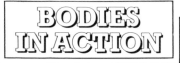

build up over the weeks and months if you exercise regularly but this level has to be sustained if you are to continue enjoying its benefits. Even after a short period of inactivity your physical condition can be affected so you cannot sit back and decrease your level of exercise when you reach a certain degree of fitness. Even if you have never enjoyed competitive sports and do not think of yourself as being an athletic person, you will be surprised at how enjoyable physical activity can be, and at how much stamina and athletic ability you really have. Most keep-fit routines and physical jerks are very boring and it is important to choose a sport or physical activity that will suit you and satisfy your requirements – for example, your age, figure, temperament, natural ability and personal preferences. The most important thing is to enjoy what you are doing and not to regard exercise as a tedious chore, a physical medicine that you have to take because it 'is good for you'. If you find swimming monotonous and boring, then try running or cycling instead or supplement it with aerobic dancing or surfing or whatever you fancy. You are more likely to stick to an exercise routine and make it an indispensable part of your life if you enjoy doing it. For more advice on choosing the right exercise, see page 56.

Your choice will probably be determined also by how competitive you are and whether you enjoy exercising alone or in the company of other people. Some people prefer to jog or cycle on their own and set themselves new targets to beat, competing against themselves. Others like to work-out or exercise with other exercise-conscious people for social and moral support, or to compete against other players and sportsmen and women on the tennis court, the athletics track or elsewhere. Most sports and activities can be as individual or as competitive as you wish and you will have to design your personal fitness programme around these requirements. If you are naturally self-conscious or shy you may prefer to exercise alone until you have the new physical confidence to mix with other like-minded people. On the other hand, there's safety in numbers and you may feel less no-

ticeable and more confident in a crowd of people exercising together. Exercising means different things to different people and we each have to discover for ourselves what is best for us and the personal benefits and experiences that it can bestow.

Physical benefits

The physical benefits of regular exercise have been debated recently in the general press but most doctors agree that exercise can make a significant contribution to our general health and well-being, both physically and psychologically, and that most people would benefit if they stepped up their levels of physical activity. Regular exercise brings about marked physiological changes and improvements in our normal body functioning, including increased muscle strength which may improve general posture and prevent or reduce back pain, and help create a stronger heart and lungs. Aerobic exercise (see page 62) in the presence of oxygen can improve the transport of oxygenated blood around our bodies, making more oxygen available for energy. An increase in the number of enzymes in our muscles heightens their ability to extract oxygen from the blood, whereas a greater density of capillaries in the muscles increases the supply of blood. Increased numbers of capillaries in the arteries mean that should a blockage occur, blood can flow through another area to supply the heart and thus the risk of heart attack is decreased.

As the heart grows stronger and larger, it can pump greater amounts of oxygenated blood to the muscles with fewer beats and less effort and your resting heart rate is lowered too. What previously necessitated a heart beat of, say, 170 beats a minute now takes only 150 beats a minute, and the strain on the cardiovascular system is reduced. When you exercise, your heart has to work harder than usual to process more blood to supply the demand from your muscles for energy. If you are unfit, your heart will have to beat very hard

A jog or walk in the country in your free time or at the weekend will help keep you active and fit. Use these times to supplement your other exercise and share them with your husband or a friend for company.

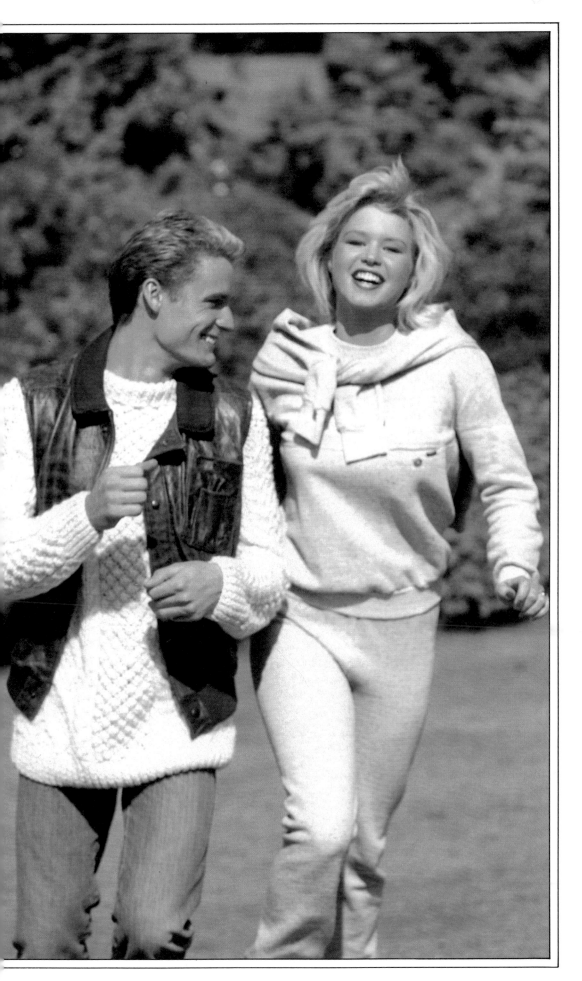

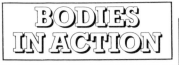

indeed and you may become out of breath and suffer slight physical discomfort, but as your general fitness improves and your heart grows stronger, it will pump blood more efficiently and easily and work less hard to perform even more difficult tasks as you push your body harder.

Researchers have found a strong relationship between the level of regular physical activity and the incidence of heart disease, and it appears that cardiovascular function is most poor among inactive people of all age groups with weak muscles. Regular exercise is an important weapon in preventing heart disease, particularly if it is combined with a well-balanced diet which is low in sugar and fats (see last chapter). Although exercise cannot influence cholesterol levels in the blood, it does appear to lower the concentration of blood fats, or triglycerides, which may block the coronary arteries. It also seems to increase high-density lipoprotein levels which are inversely related to the incidence of heart disease. Thus inactive people in sedentary jobs who do not exercise in their leisure time and eat a diet that is high in fats are more likely to suffer from heart disease at some time in their lives than are physically active people. As more and more people embark on a programme of regular exercise and improve their diets, scientists will be able to monitor their progress and discover even more about the effects of exercise on health.

Many rehabilitation programmes for people convalescing from heart, respiratory and muscular diseases now include exercise training, jogging, running and swimming in particular, and there are even accomplished marathon runners who took up running after suffering a heart attack and are now competing in major sporting events.

When your body is in good working order, you will find that you have more stamina and a higher physical working capacity so that you can perform any given task with less effort. Your physical involvement in life is increased and your daily life can be enriched by your enhanced capacity for physical and mental energy. If you can establish now a positive exercise programme which you enjoy, and

can sustain it throughout your middle years and even into old age your chances of good health will be improved enormously. However, a word of warning before you dash out and overdo it: if you are significantly overweight or are over 35 years of age, then have a medical check-up first to ensure that there are no medical reasons why you should not exercise. This is a good idea if you have a family background of heart disease, or if you drink or smoke heavily. It is always wise to take precautions and seek expert advice if you have any doubts about your health. If you are reasonably strong and active, however, then go ahead and providing you take it gradually and build up slowly, you should not experience any problems. If, however, you experience persistent chest pains or dizziness, then stop at once and make an appointment to see your doctor before you continue exercising.

Of course, not all exercises are good for all-over and cardiovascular conditioning and endurance. Whereas some aerobic exercises, like swimming, running, cycling, rowing and cross-country skiing, use nearly all the muscles in your body and help you to develop muscular strength and suppleness, general fitness and greater heart-lung capacity, some forms of exercise, such as badminton, tennis and squash, give short bursts of energy only and strengthen specific groups of muscles. In fact, reliance on these exercises alone may be dangerous rather than beneficial to health. How many times have you heard people claim that they are fit because they play squash twice a week or enjoy a knock-about on the tennis court or football pitch at weekends? But these people may be deluding themselves and it is only when they go out running or cycling and try to sustain a rhythmic aerobic exercise over a given period of, say, 30 minutes that they realise how unfit they really are. Casual exercise can put unnecessary strain on the heart which it is under-conditioned to cope with, and the short bursts of energy

Badminton and tennis (inset) are fun to play and will get you mobile and supple. You can learn how at sports centres and clubs where expert tuition in the game, serving, footwork and basic strokes is usually available.

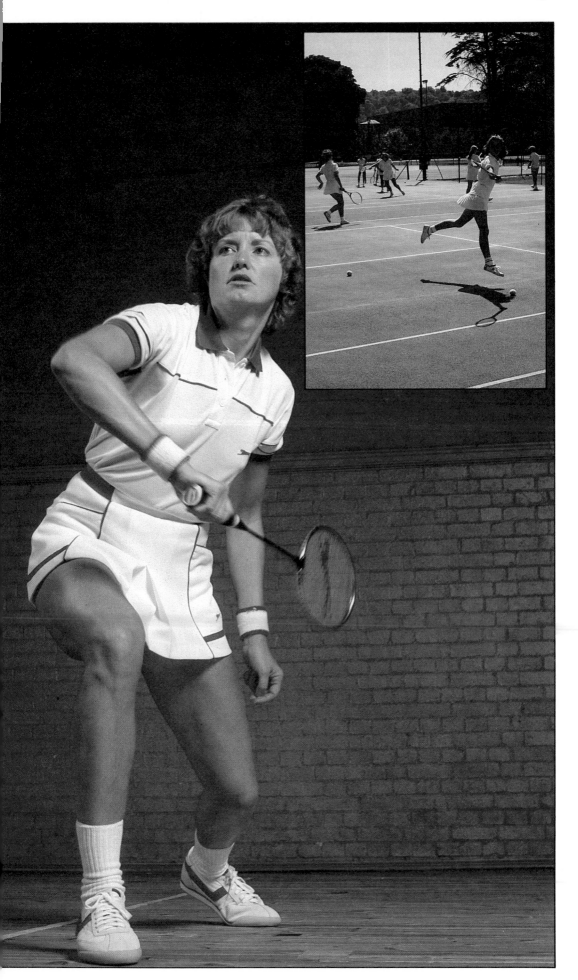

needed in a game of squash or tennis may put excessive pressure on muscles too and lead to strains and tears. This is particularly true in the case of sedentary office workers and housewives who play infrequently for social reasons.

The only safe and effective way to get really fit and feel the physical benefits is to exercise regularly and rhythmically for 20 to 30 minutes at least three times a week. You can supplement this healthier aerobic exercise with a sport such as tennis to develop speed, agility and suppleness, for as your heart and muscles get stronger you will be better fitted to deal with the physical demands of other sports and less vulnerable to injury. Stretching exercises are also good for developing muscular flexibility, and even some weight-lifting for strength. So design your exercise programme around a combination of the sports and exercises that you enjoy.

Losing weight

Many people take up regular exercise because they want to lose weight or, at least, control their weight and maintain it at an acceptable level. If exercise is used to supplement a weight-reducing diet, then it can be very effective indeed as it increases your metabolic rate and helps burn up calories, particularly very vigorous sustained exercise, such as running or swimming. However, exercise alone will not reduce weight and it is no good running for 30 minutes if you devour cream buns and chocolate bars with gay abandon afterwards. Some people find that their weight stays pretty steady during the first few weeks of an exercise programme, although when they look in the mirror they appear slimmer and firmer as their bodies become stronger and more supple.

Everybody responds differently and even if weight loss is slow at first, do not despair as all your hard work *will* produce results and a slimmer figure, although it may take longer for your body to respond to increased exercise than it does for

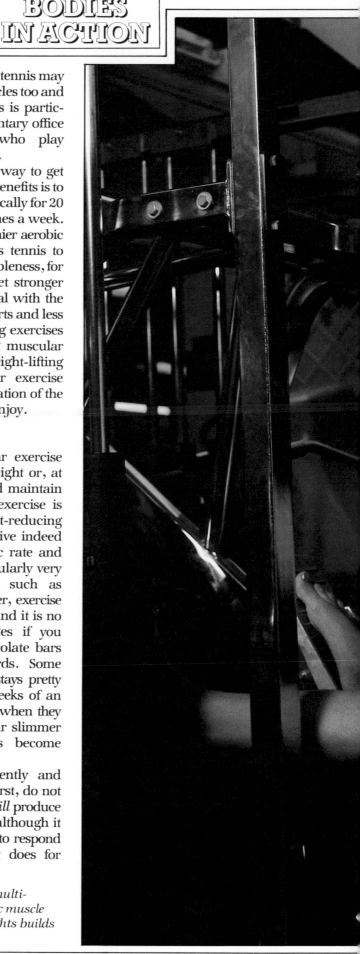

Many gyms now have their own multi-exercisers for working-out specific muscle groups. The resistance of the weights builds up both strength and endurance.

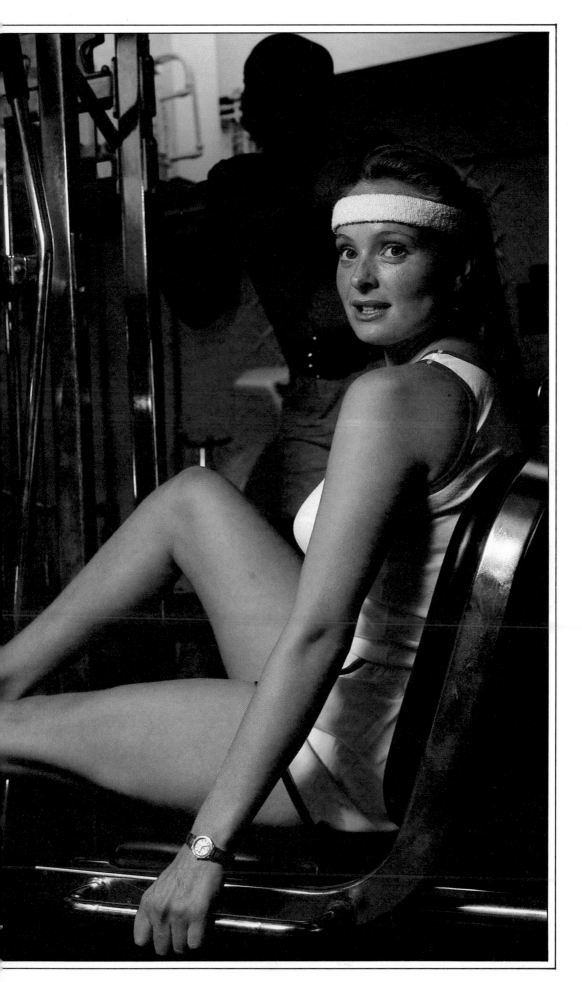

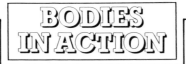

some other people. Persevere and any unsightly bulges will disappear as you burn up fat and develop firm muscle tissue. Nor is there any need to worry about building up large, rippling muscles. Many woman excuse themselves from exercise on the grounds that it will make them muscle-bound and unfeminine. However, male hormones, notably testosterone, are necessary to build up large muscles and even weight-training in moderation will not cause you to become incredibly muscular. Instead, your body will become stronger, firmer and leaner and you will feel more attractive as a result, as well as fitter and healthier.

Another reason for not exercising that is often put forward is that it increases your appetite, thus causing you to eat more and put on weight as a result. But scientific studies in both Britain and the United States have found that an increase in exercise does not appear to be accompanied by a compensatory rise in appetite. Thus you do not need to increase your calorie intake and eat more just because you are burning up more calories through exercise. On the contrary, research findings show that regular exercise may actually decrease appetite as it helps prevent a drop in blood sugar levels which gives rise to hunger; it speeds up the transit time of food through your digestive system; and it increases your metabolic rate in such a way that your body makes more efficient

Explosive sports such as sprinting fall within the anaerobic sphere of activity. Anaerobics call for great bursts of speed and power in which the oxygen supplied to the muscles is insufficient for their needs.

use of the nutrients you take in and thus you need less food for energy.

Slimming regimes in the past have under-valued the role of exercise in weight reduction, relying heavily instead on dietary control and even the use of appetite-suppressant drugs. But if you slim solely by these means and do not exercise, you are likely to weaken your muscles and lose valuable muscular tissue which may turn to fat when you stop dieting. Unless you exercise regularly, you are probably going to regain some, if not all, of the weight you have lost, particularly if you do not control your diet rigorously. However, the stimulating effect of exercise on metabolism can persist throughout the day even after you have stopped exercising, raising your metabolic rate in such a way that you lose more calories than would be expected for the level of physical exertion undertaken.

In a society where more than 40 per cent of the adult population are judged to be obese, it is more important than ever that we get fit and slim through exercise and sport. Being overweight is not healthy and may trigger off many medical disorders and diseases, including diabetes, heart disease and abdominal problems. Exercise is an effective and enjoyable way of controlling your diet and reducing your risk of falling prey to these modern 'affluent' diseases. Although you can half-starve yourself on a trendy diet and emerge a lot thinner, it does not make you fitter or healthier, probably the reverse, and the weight will soon return if you do not take steps to control it. Sensible diet and regular exercise are the most effective ways to lose weight and keep it off for good

Remember that if you are heavily overweight to check with your doctor before you exercise strenuously, and if you are on a very low-calorie regime, then don't exercise too vigorously or you may feel weak and dizzy. Exercise caution and common sense.

Staying young

There are no age barriers to exercise and you are never too old to start as many older people are finding out. It is a pity that some people wait until they are in their fifties or sixties before they discover the benefits and pleasure that exercise can bring. Of course, the sooner you start the greater the benefits throughout your life and the better your chances of staying youthful and healthy and avoiding many degenerative diseases, especially in late middle and old age.

Most people who are physically active and sporting in their youth, tend to decrease their exercise levels as they get older and become more sedentary in middle age. There are many reasons for this: they may have less leisure time for sport as they marry and have families and their jobs become more demanding; they

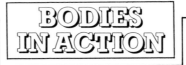

may associate sport and exercise with being young and consider themselves too old; or they may retire after an injury and not resume their exercise when they are fully recovered. They are foolish, whatever their reasons, as regular exercise can keep your body strong, muscular and flexible, and the cardiovascular conditioning that comes from aerobic activity can make you less vulnerable to heart disease and a whole host of other age-related illnesses.

Exercise can actually delay the ageing process in our bodies and help retain a youthful appearance and levels of energy. It can help prevent muscles shrinking as we grow older, and keep skin healthy and firm with fewer wrinkles and age-lines. A firm, slim body with strong muscles and healthy, glowing skin is more youthful than an old, flabby one. Even if you start exercising after many years of inactivity, muscle power and cardiovascular fitness can be restored and maintained, and you will feel fitter and healthier than you have done for years.

As your level of inactivity increases you become more prone to a whole range of debilitating diseases, especially if you are under stress or very elderly. Some inactive people look old in their forties whereas some active sixty- and seventy-year-olds look young and sprightly. Older people taking up exercise should choose something regular and rhythmic such as swimming, jogging or walking. Swift, jerky movements might be injurious to stiff joints and weakened muscles. It is better to build up fitness slowly and safely – just increasing the distance you walk every day gradually can help.

Health, fitness and beauty are not the exclusive preserve of the young and you can look good and feel fit at any age. Your genetic make-up, your diet, skin-care routine, environment, level of exercise and the amount of stress you are subjected to can all determine the speed at which you age. Stress, in particular, can accelerate the ageing process as it depletes your body of its energy and resistance. Likewise, an inactive lifestyle can cause bones and muscles to weaken and shrink and this, in turn, affects the functioning of the endocrine system and the production of hormones in the body for sustaining vitality. Therefore it is terribly important to exercise regularly and keep your body strong and healthy so that you can enjoy a more active later life.

Is exercise unfeminine?

Exercise has long been considered a male activity in which women tend to figure only as second-class citizens because they are not as strong or as fast as men are with their superior muscular make-up. For many years, sports were held to be unfeminine and unladylike, and although increasing numbers of women are now actively engaged in sport and regular exercise they are still ridiculed and criticised by some chauvinistic men. However, despite some masculine opposition, the barriers to women's participation in sport are now crumbling and exercise is a big exciting growth area for women who no longer feel self-conscious or shy about putting on a tracksuit, leotard or shorts and taking part in energetic exercise.

Traditionally the weaker sex, women are now proving on the athletics track, in the gym, the swimming pool and many other areas just how fit and strong they can be, and they have excelled themselves in endurance events, such as marathon and ultra-distance running and the triathlon. Until a few years ago, only ball-games, such as tennis, hockey, netball and badminton, and short explosive athletic events were deemed suitable for women – they were considered too weak and delicate for endurance sports. In fact, the first Olympics women's marathon will be staged in 1984 at the Los Angeles games. Now women are setting new records in a wide range of sports as they dispel the myth that exercise is unfeminine once and for all.

Today's modern attractive woman is independent, self-assured, strong, fit and healthy, a far cry from the fragile, ornamental woman of the past. Although she is well aware of her femininity, she is

Skiing and horse-riding are both good forms of exercise as well as great ways of spending a holiday. Both these healthy sports will strengthen your leg muscles and get you out in the open air and the sunshine.

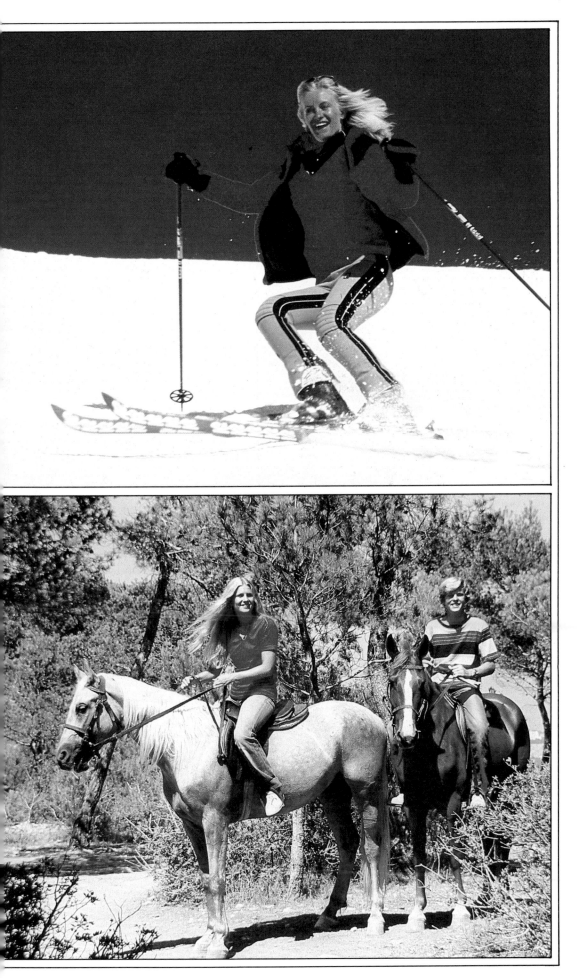

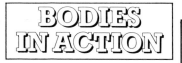
equally conscious of the benefits that regular exercise can bring and she aims to stay at the peak of her physical potential for maximum fitness and the realisation of her unique feminine qualities. True health and beauty came from within oneself and are derived from a general feeling of physical and mental well-being and the development of one's full creative potential as a woman.

Women are traditionally good at supporting and caring for others and accommodating and adjusting their lives to the needs and demands of their husbands, families and friends. They are socialised into trusting and relying on men and hiding behind their passive feminine roles. Unlike men, whose cultural role is to be strong, independent, forceful, decisive and active, women have long been considered as weak, dependent, vacillating, accommodating, gentle and submissive. However, feminine roles are changing in our highly technological society and many women have to fulfil the role of successful career woman as well as wife and mother. As matrimonial breakdown and one-parent familes become commonplace, more and more women are assuming the role of head of the household too and all the responsibilities it carries with it.

Today's woman has to be stronger, more self-assertive, an initiator of action, not just a passive onlooker or assistant. She has found her ability to act and express herself intellectually, emotionally and physically without losing her quintessential femininity.

Many women have discovered that regular exercise has given them a new sense of purpose and self-awareness as they achieve new goals and realise their physical capabilities. Having been brought up to be under-achievers and naturally cautious about pushing themselves to their limits in any activities, they are making exercise an integral part of their lives and giving physical fitness top priority as they become more confident and discover the joy that physical movement can bring. We all moved naturally as children but as we get older we become more self-conscious about our bodies, and many women are afraid to start an exercise plan for fear of looking foolish and being laughed at by their family, neighbours and friends. If you are shy or

An economical means of transport, cycling will also make you aerobically fit. Make it a regular feature of your life in order to stay fit and healthy. Cycle to work or the shops.

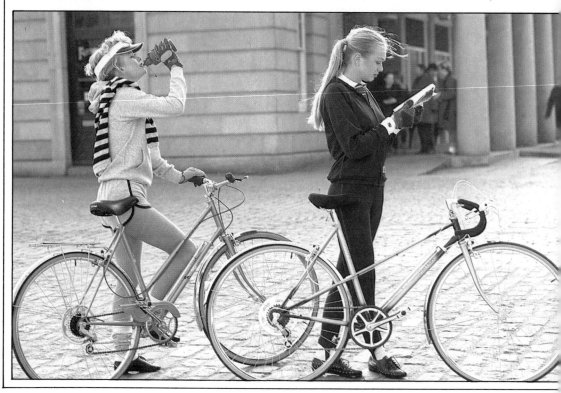

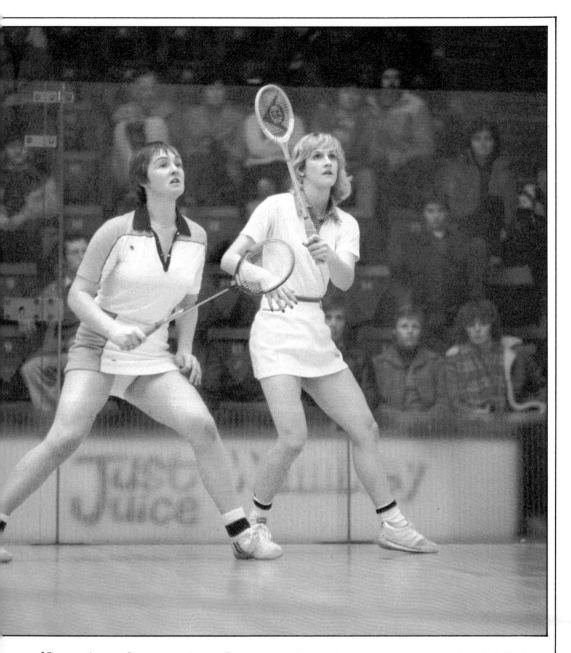

Squash requires great speed and skill if played correctly. Here, Lisa Opie plays Felicity Hargreaves.

self-conscious, then exercise at home or go out running or cycling early in the morningwhile the streets are still relatively empty. As you become fitter and trimmer, your confidence will grow, you will feel proud of your new slim body and increased energy and vitality, and your shyness will disappear. Teaming up with a friend for moral support is a good idea for some women, and you can have fun sharing the discovery of exercise together and motivating each other to do better as a friendly rivalry develops.

It takes determination and guts to embark on a fitness plan, especially after many years of inactivity. Athletic ability is not so essential as feeling fitter and healthier and creating a new individual role for yourself. Just do your own thing –

all you need are character, determination, self-discipline and patience. Getting fit is hard work and there are no easy short-cuts but the benefits will make it all worthwhile. You need not be naturally aggressive and competitive to get fit – there are many forms of exercise that you can practise alone. Walking, running, cycling, swimming, cross-country skiing are excellent all-round conditioners that can be enjoyed in a non-competitive way.

Some women may worry that making a commitment to regular exercise may encroach on their family responsibilities and they may end up neglecting their children or husband. It is hard work to run a home, a job and a family and to make time to exercise as well, but in the long run it is worthwhile for the increased enjoyment and fulfilment it brings and the long-term health and beauty benefits. Far from feeling tired as a result of regular exercise, you will find that you have more energy and stamina for tackling your everyday life. Because you will not tire so easily, you will be less irritable and stressful and will enjoy your family relationships more and play a more active role at home and at work. Your husband and family may laugh at first at mum setting out around the park in her track-suit, or working-out in her leotard at home or in the gym, but they will soon appreciate your new figure, increased vitality and sense of enjoyment and fun.

Exercise can bestow other physical benefits on women, too. Women who exercise regularly tend to suffer less from menstrual pain and cramping, and steady rhythmic exercise may even reduce and relieve these symptoms. Regular exercise before and during pregnancy increases general fitness and oxygenisation of your blood. During labour your muscles need plenty of oxygen, like those of an athlete in training, and if you are fit and strong with supple elastic muscles, your labour is likely to be trouble-free and quicker than that of an unfit woman. In fact, the stronger your muscles, the shorter and easier the delivery.

Designing your own personal fitness programme

When planning your personal fitness pro-gramme bear in mind that there are several different kinds of exercise which are beneficial for different reasons. They are usually classified as being aerobic, anaerobic or isotonic. To become really fit, you should aim to include a combi-nation of these different exercise forms in your plan. For example, anaerobics can train your body for powerful bursts of speed and strength; aerobics helps you develop cardiovascular fitness and endu-rance; isotonics moves joints and stretches out muscles for suppleness and flexibility.

Fitness means being supple, strong, energetic and having stamina and mo-

Planning your own exercise programme allows you to choose the sports and activities you enjoy, whether it's running (below) or working out (right). Be sure to include some aerobic exercise as well as stretching and games such as tennis or squash to ensure maximum overall fitness.

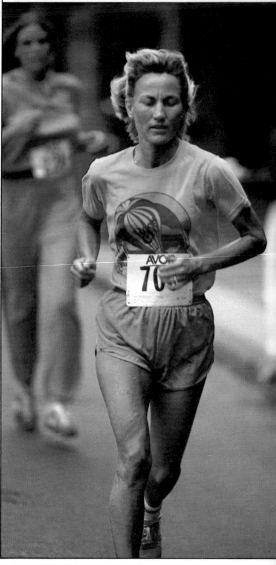

How does your sport rate?

Sport/exercise	Calories burned per hour
Badminton	250
Cycling	350
Dancing	300
Jogging	500
Running	800
Skiing	700
Skipping	300
Squash	600
Swimming	400
Surfing	300
Tennis	350
Water-skiing	300
Wind-surfing	350
Walking briskly	400

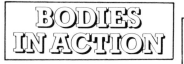

bility. Your fitness programme can incorporate different forms of exercise and sports to promote these qualities as well as yoga for tranquillity and peace of mind, and golf or walking, say, for relaxation. The choice is yours — just choose the exercises that interest you and that you enjoy doing and devise a programme around them so that you start off by exercising at least three times a week for 30 minutes in each session, plus a warming-up and warming-down phase before and after exercise (page 94). In addition, you can introduce stretching sessions two or three times a week of about 15 minutes' duration to develop maximum flexibility of muscles. Well toned and flexible muscles will utilise oxygen more efficiently for energy during exercise, and are also less likely to become strained or injured than are tight, tense muscles. Stretching before and after strenuous exercise will also ease out muscles and reduce the tension and stiffness experienced by many people who are unused to exercise. Always stretch muscles out slowly — the long, slow stretch is far more beneficial than short, jerky stretches which can damage muscles.

Plan your programme so that you set aside a regular time for exercise each week, choosing the time of day that suits you best. There are no set rules about this — it is a matter for your personal preference and timetable. Thus some people like to exercise first thing in the morning before they go to work, whereas others prefer to utilise their lunch-hour or the evenings after work. It is your decision, but make sure that you make a regular date with exercise that is unbreakable. It will soon become an established part of your weekly or daily routine and you will feel disappointed and even guilty if you miss a session. It is sometimes a good idea to share your fitness commitment with your family or friends so that it becomes a social affair and there is more pressure on you not to miss a training session. It is harder to cry off then than if you exercise by yourself.

When you start out, exercise on alternate days initially giving yourself a day of rest in between sessions for your body to recover. It may feel a little stiff at first until your muscles grow accustomed to the new, unfamiliar movements through which they are being pushed. However, the stiffness should last for only a day and this will soon pass as the weeks go by and you become fitter and stronger. It should be no more than a feeling of slight discomfort. If it is really painful and you find that you can hardly move for several days, then you have been overdoing it and you should cut back on your training accordingly. There is no doubt that exercise will be hard and difficult until you start to feel more relaxed and supple and experience the benefits that true fitness can bring, but when the first signs appear it will all seem worthwhile. Build it up slowly and gradually and be patient until your body becomes conditioned to your new exercise regime. Do not risk forfeiting the progress you have made by overdoing your training and then having to miss a few days through stiffness or injury. After exercising always take a bath or shower to cool down and take the sting out of tired muscles. Allocate enough time for this and don't rush your exercise to fit it in — it should always be relaxed and enjoyable.

Remember when devising your programme that unless you really enjoy exercising you will never be able to stick to any exercise plan. Although we are brought up to believe in the old puritan work ethic that anything worth achieving does not come easily and that we must all suffer a little to accomplish our goals, exercise should be enjoyable and fun. It should make us feel good as well as doing us good, and as the initial aches and pains fade away and you get fitter and more proficient, you should enjoy it more. If

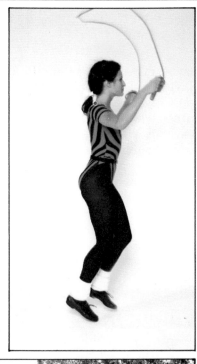

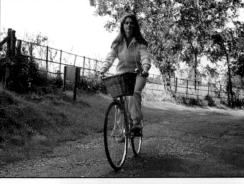

Skipping, cycling and running are all
different forms of aerobic exercise which
will condition your cardiovascular
system and make you fit and strong.
They are all performed at a regular
rhythmical pace and should be
sustained for at least 20 minutes if you
are to receive any real benefit. Practise
them three or four times every week.

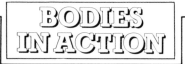
you don't enjoy it you may end up feeling guilty and depressed instead of excited and invigorated, and you should think about changing to a different form of exercise that will meet your personal requirements and preferences better. Build the pleasure principle into your exercise routine and you will feel satisfied and revitalised afterwards. Exercise is challenging and exhilarating, but it should be rewarding too. You should feel in good spirits, even though you may be slightly fatigued afterwards. Do not let the challenge of exercise fade away but make it a habit that is impossible to break.

You will know that you are getting fit when you tire less easily, breathe more naturally, have greater stamina and flexibility. Your friends and family may even comment on how well and healthy you look. You will appear slimmer and firmer when you look at yourself in the mirror. At this point, you can congratulate yourself on your progress so far, but don't let it

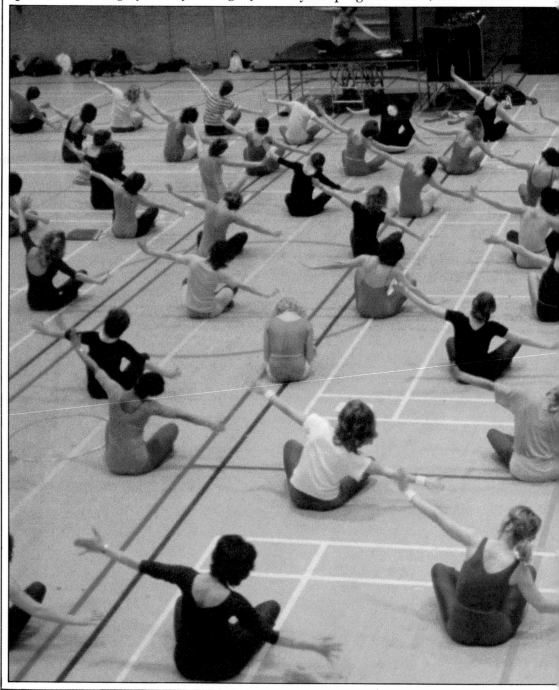

lapse because now you have to maintain this newly acquired level of fitness and make it part of your life. This is not difficult as you will come to enjoy the benefits it brings — you will feel less tired and more energetic, you will sleep more easily and soundly, you will be better equipped to cope with stress, you will have greater powers of concentration for tackling work, you will look slimmer and feel healthier. With all these plus factors, how could you possibly stop exercising?

Some people find that it is a good idea to keep a record of their progress in the early weeks — a sort of training diary so that they can check up on how they are coming along. It is heartening to look back on the improvements you have made as the weeks go by and to compare your ever-growing sense of fitness with the early difficult sessions when health and fitness were still elusive unknown quantities. Buy a notebook and jot down the date, the type of exercise undertaken, the time spent

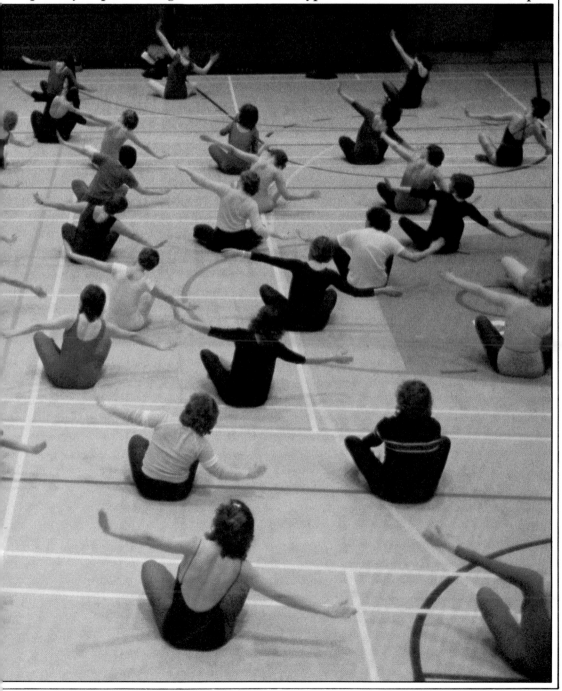

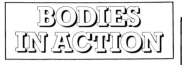
and how you felt, along with details of your weight and pulse rates too if you wish (see below). This could motivate you to set yourself new goals and challenges and will encourage you not to miss an exercise session.

Before you start exercising, you should stop and analyse your personal level of fitness and ask yourself: 'How fit am I?' For instance:

★ **Do I get out of breath running for the bus or charging upstairs?**
★ **Can I walk four miles or run one mile without feeling breathless and discomfort, or even pain?**
★ **Can I touch my toes?**
★ **Can I do 10 sit-ups or press-ups without cheating?**
★ **Am I more than 3.5kg/7lb over-weight?**
★ **Do I tire easily?**

If you are honest with yourself, you may be suprised at how unfit you really are. So make a commitment now and plan your programme around the following kinds of exercise.

Aerobics

This is the most beneficial exercise of all for achieving overall health and fitness. Instead of exercising the body part by part, it involves the entire body in total movement, which is both steady and rhythmical. All sustained, rhythmical exercise forms that use large muscle groups fall within this category. They include distance running, cycling, swimming, cross-country skiing, rowing, and even sustained skipping and really long walks at a brisk pace. It was Dr Kenneth Cooper who showed the value of aerobic exercise when he used aerobics to rehabilitate patients who had suffered heart attacks in the late 1960s. He discovered that medically controlled physical exercise restored them to full health and many achieved a level of physical fitness that they had never experienced previously. His book *Aerobics* became a bestseller, and a great deal of research

has been done since then into the value of aerobic exercise.

The basic principle underlying aerobic exercise is that the oxygen utilised by the body is roughly sufficient to meet its energy requirements. Thus oxygen is supplied to the muscles for energy and movement at the same rate at which it is used and you never get into oxygen debt — when you feel weak and gasping for more oxygen. When you are aerobically fit, your body uses oxygen more efficiently, and your cardiovascular system (heart, lungs and circulatory system) are strengthened. You have greater endurance and muscle power, your lung capacity is increased, your arteries become more elastic and your heart becomes stronger and enlarged. Your metabolism also improves so that waste products, toxins and excess fat are removed more easily, leaving you fitter and healthier.

So the aerobic body is stronger and more efficient, with greater resistance to heart disease and other degenerative illnesses. Aerobic exercise has to be built up gradually, especially if you have led a very sedentary life. When you are aerobically unfit, your cells and muscles will be short of oxygen and you will not get an adequate supply when you exercise. You will feel breathless running upstairs perhaps or swimming a couple of lengths of the pool. To achieve full aerobic fitness, you must increase your heart rate to a training level and sustain this level over a given period of time, say, 20 to 30 minutes at least three times a week. Most adults have a resting pulse rate of 60 to 80 beats per minute but this increases when we exercise and put our bodies under pressure. The heart has to beat harder and faster to supply oxygenated blood to the muscles to meet their increased energy requirements. You can determine your training level by a simple calculation. For your maximum level, subtract your age from 200, and for your minimum level subtract your age from 170. Your optimum

A game of golf is a gentle, relaxing form of exercise and a good way of meeting other people. Although it is essentially a game of technique, walking the course gets you fit and it can supplement other sports.

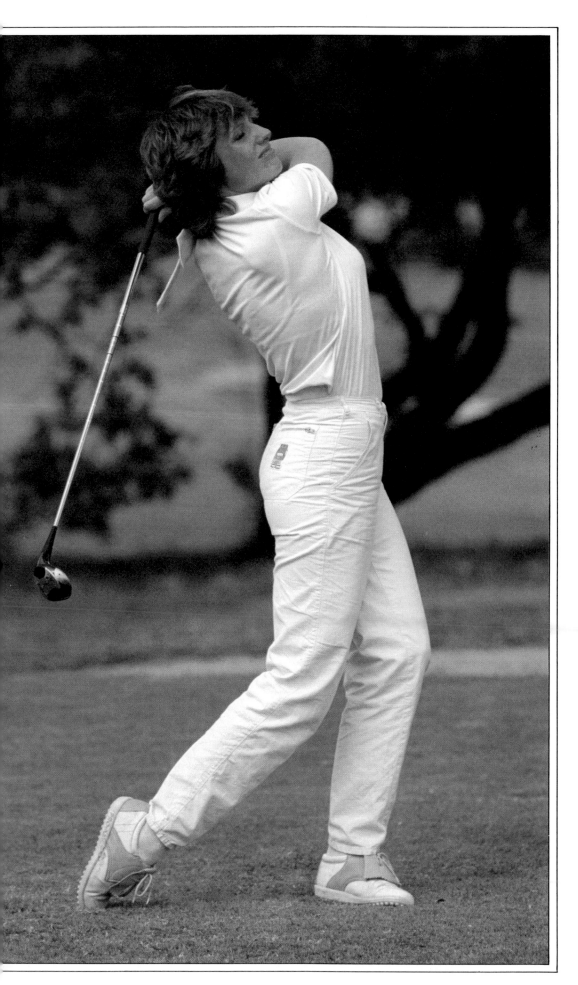

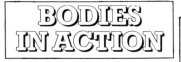

training level will fall somewhere between these two figures. Thus if you are 30, your training level will be in the 140-170 beats per minute range. Take your pulse by pressing your wrist on the thumb side for 15 seconds and then multiply by four to find your pulse rate per minute. Practise taking your pulse before exercising to find out your resting rate, and then during exercise to see whether you are performing at your training level. If it is lower than your minimum permissible level, then you are not exercising hard enough. If, on the other hand, it is higher than your maximum permissible level, you are overdoing it and should slow down.

Exercising aerobically pushes up your heart rate until it is between 70 and 85 per cent of its maximum capacity. As you become aerobically fit and your heart gets stronger, your resting heart rate will be lower and your heart will pump more blood with each beat, and therefore more blood will reach the tissues and cells. Oxygen transfer to the bloodstream and transport around the body will improve as the number and size of the blood vessels are increased, and the strain on the cardiovascular system is decreased. Regular aerobic exercise will make your body so efficient that you will have more energy for other tasks and your heart will develop its own built-in protection against stress and strain.

Anaerobics

This form of exercise is the opposite of aerobics. Instead of steady rhythmic exercise, anaerobics are performed at high speed so that the oxygen supply to the working muscles is insufficient to meet their energy requirements. Therefore effort cannot be maintained for long as the body gets into oxygen debt. However, these explosive bursts of energy do help to develop muscular power and strength and are a useful training supplement to aerobic exercise in order to process oxygen even more efficiently. Sprinting, some gymnastics and even a vigorous game of squash all fall into the category of anaerobic exercise. Some people, of course, are more suited to anaerobic activities by virtue of their muscular make-up. Our muscular system is composed of a mixture of slow-

twitch and fast-twitch fibres and the degree to which we possess either of these types of fibres influences our athletic performance and the sort of exercise at which we excel. A preponderance of fast-twitch fibres indicates that you are better suited to fast anaerobic events, whereas a larger number of slow-twitch fibres means you will perform better in aerobic endurance exercise. To determine your muscle make-up, compare your performances in different sports and exercises. If you can run, cycle or swim without undue distress for 20 to 30 minutes, then there is a good chance that your slow fibres are dominant, but if you find it easier to summon up great bursts of energy and speed for a really fast sprint, then some form of anaerobic training is probably more suitable. Most people tend to be aerobically orientated and will benefit from regular endurance exercise. This is probably a good thing as anaerobic exercise cannot be endured for long enough to benefit your heart and lungs and must be combined with some aerobic training to produce real fitness.

Isotonics

These exercises help you to develop muscular strength and flexibility. They include stretching exercises (calisthenics), yoga and weightlifting. Many of the new work-out classes and California stretch routines feature these exercises. Although they cannot give overall fitness and cardiovascular endurance, these exercises will help make your muscles more supple and elastic as they are based on the rhythmic movement of muscles and joints. They should be performed slowly and rhythmically for greater stretch and to ease out any tension. When you start a course of stretching exercises, you will probably be surprised at how out of condition you are. Your muscles will feel sore and stiff afterwards but the ache will soon go as they become toned up and conditioned. Little by little, you will be

Womens' athletics are becoming fiercely competitive at all levels as runners strive to set new records. Of course you don't have to compete on the track — you can just jog round the roads or run cross-country.

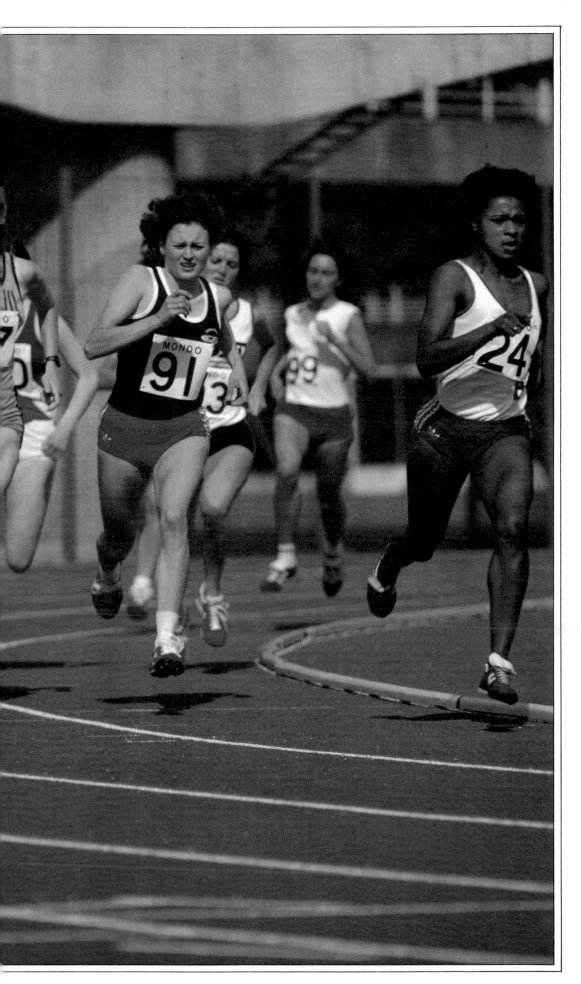

able to extend your muscles even further and you will move more gracefully.

You may not burn up a lot of calories but your body will assume its natural proportions in time and you will look leaner and firmer with a stronger, healthier body. The exercises are particularly effective if combined with an aerobic exercise regime. Incorporate them within your warm-up before you start your aerobic activity to take the tension out of tired muscles. That way, you can avoid many common athletic injuries and run, cycle, swim or ski faster and more easily. If you play games such as tennis or squash, stretching exercises will help your overall mobility and flexibility on the court. Develop a routine and stretch to music if it helps you to concentrate better and establish a flowing rhythm. Choose a disco or pop record. You might find it useful to alternate days of stretching and

isotonics with other forms of exercise, especially aerobics which need be performed only three to five times per week. That way, you will get really fit and healthy.

Working with weights also comes under the heading of isotonics as it involves the lengthening and shortening of muscles to build up strength. Many women are now using weights as part of their regular exercise routine. Used properly, weights will help you develop strength and endurance and a firmer, slimmer looking body. Weights make your body work harder and are good for firming your sides and bustline. They can also be strapped to the ankles for toning up leg muscles.

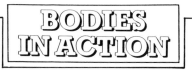

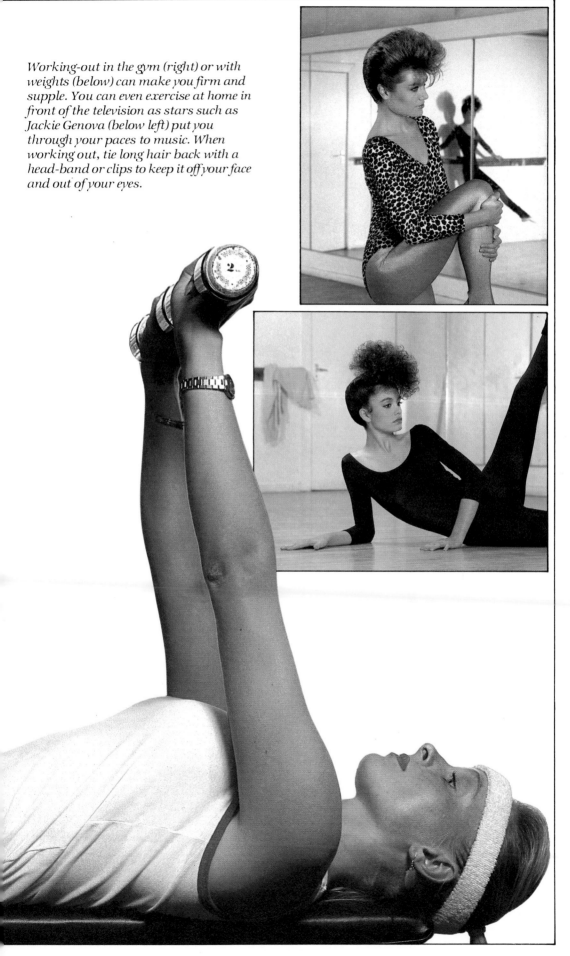

Working-out in the gym (right) or with weights (below) can make you firm and supple. You can even exercise at home in front of the television as stars such as Jackie Genova (below left) put you through your paces to music. When working out, tie long hair back with a head-band or clips to keep it off your face and out of your eyes.

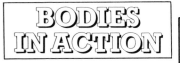

Exercise safety code

Before you rush out and start exercising, study the following safety guide. It will tell you the safest way to get fit and how to take the right precautions for avoiding injury. Most injuries occur as a result of over-zealous exercise or thoughtlessness so exercise a little caution and do it the safe way.

Never exercise immediately after eating. Wait at least two hours after a meal in order to avoid stomach ache and cramps.

Do not exercise if you have a fever or virus infection. They will affect your performance and may cause muscles, joints, your heart or respiratory system to become inflamed and the condition will worsen. Wait until you are feeling better and then gradually build up your exercises to their previous level as you get stronger.

If you are very overweight, have a history of high blood pressure, diabetes or heart disease, or are over 35 years old, have a medical check-up before embarking on an exercise programme.

Never exercise in really hot weather. It is debilitating and you may become dehydrated. Wait until the cool of the evening or exercise early in the morning or inside in an air-conditioned environment.

Always build up gradually and slowly at your chosen exercise. It may take several weeks before you begin to feel any real benefits so do not try to overdo it. Be patient and the results will soon become manifest as you feel fitter and trimmer. Remember to train, not strain, and listen to your body and the messages it communicates to you. At first it will be hard and your body will feel heavy and sluggish, but as you persevere it will gradually become lighter and your movements more fluid and graceful. As exercise becomes more effortless, you will get fitter and healthier.

Always warm-up before exercising (see page 94 for basic warm-up exercises and routines). A proper warm-up will get your muscles accustomed to increased activity and reduce the risk of stiffness later. Although you may feel like exercising, your body might not, so get it used to the idea gradually before you launch into your jog, swim, a game of tennis, squash, cycling or whatever. Warming-up releases tension in the muscles and stretches them out ready for action. It also helps your maximum oxygen capacity and gets your heart beating faster so that you are prepared for action.

7

If the exercise becomes painful, stop and stretch gently and slowly to ease out the pain and tension in sore muscles — it may only be stiffness. If it continues, however, stop exercising at once and rest. Likewise if you feel giddy, faint, out of breath or sick. If the condition persists after adequate rest, consult your doctor.

8

Always wear the right clothing — something loose, comfortable and non-constricting is best. Tight jeans and tops are not suitable as they inhibit freedom of movement and put strain on the body. Wear a loose tracksuit, shorts and T-shirt or sweatshirt, or a leotard and tights. Wrap up warmly in cold weather to prevent muscles cramping and becoming tight and sore. This makes them more prone to injury.

Stretching before you exercise will help reduce the risk of injury and ease out tense or stiff muscles. Always stretch gently and slowly, never in fast, jerky movements which might damage or even tear muscles.

9

Always cool down after any strenuous physical activity to help you relax and to allow your pulse rate to return to normal. Gentle stretching will ease out tired muscles and help prevent stiffness and soreness. Shake out your legs and arms and bend over from the hips with your arms hanging loosely down towards the floor. Lie on your back with the soles of your feet together and let your knees drop out towards the floor on either side, pressing the small of your back into the floor as you do so. Stretch out calf and hamstring muscles (see exercise on page 104) and then relax.

10

After the cool-down, relax in a warm bath or a shower to feel really refreshed and clean and warm up your tired muscles. It is sometimes a good idea to massage your leg muscles gently as you do so to release tension. Then a vigorous rub dry with a soft towel and you will feel really refreshed and invigorated.

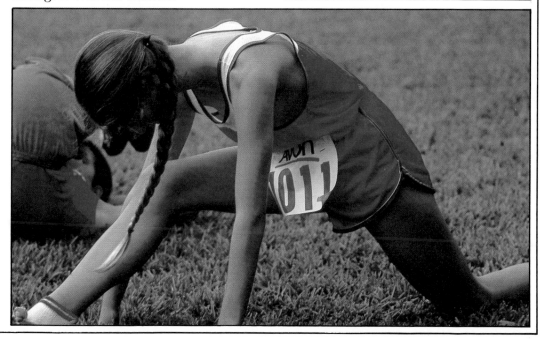

Should exercise hurt?

Although we are urged by some fitness fanatics to 'make it burn' and keep going until we can physically bear the pain no longer, exercise should not have to hurt to do us good. You do not have to pass the pain threshold or sweat profusely to benefit from exercise. Putting excessive strain on your body may, in fact, harm it and you are likely to end up with damaged muscles and ligaments. All exercise should be enjoyable, stimulating and fun. It may be demanding and challenging when you start a course of exercise and you will certainly experience some soreness and stiffness and your fair share of laboured breathing, but these symptoms will soon pass as you get fitter.

Learn to differentiate between the 'good' pains that are perfectly natural when your body is unaccustomed to an increase in physical activity and are just mildly uncomfortable, and the unacceptable warning pains that signify that you are overdoing it and should ease down before you injure yourself. Most exercises feel unfamiliar and uncomfortable at first but they will not harm you if performed properly. Do not overwork muscles until they can cope with the additional workload. Stretch them out gently without any fast, jerky movements — it is safer, more effective and less painful. Do not suffer from unnecessary injuries that are self-induced just because you have been told that exercise should hurt. It should not.

Another myth that many people still believe is that you cannot exercise aerobically without feeling breathless, tired and soaked in sweat. When this happens, you are exercising anaerobically (without oxygen) rather than aerobically (with oxygen). Exercise should always feel pleasant and comfortable. You will not receive any benefits from pushing yourself too hard and starving your muscles of adequate oxygen. You are more likely to feel breathless, giddy, faint and sick. Learn to recognise when you should stop and rest to recover your strength and breath, and only continue exercising when you feel better and fully recovered. When you are really fit and operating at your training level you should be able to hold a normal conversation as you exercise.

Sweatsuits are another means of making exercise unnecessarily tiring and uncomfortable. Their devotees claim that they will help you burn up fat, and they will certainly make you feel very wet and sticky indeed. However, medical research suggests that sweating does not aid significantly in weight loss and although you will lose body fluids while you exercise you will regain this lost weight immediately afterwards when you take in fluids as a result of feeling dehydrated and very thirsty. Far from doing you good, sweatsuits prevent normal evaporation of body heat into the air. Be sensible and exercise your heart and muscles only, *not* your sweat glands. It is safer and easier to lose weight through a controlled programme of exercise and diet.

The right gear

Your clothing and equipment for exercise and sports are important for a number of reasons. Sports equipment is now a growth industry and there are so many products and styles available that you may find it difficult to choose what suits you best. Your choice may be influenced by your budget, your individual requirements and preferences and your level of participation. Obviously it is foolish to buy a very expensive tennis racket if you play only once a month or to purchase pricy running shoes when you are just beginning a jogging programme. Use your common sense before you rush out and spend a lot of money in a fit of ill-judged enthusiasm. Remember also that expensive is not necessarily best, and that the latest fashions will cost more than last year's styles. Most people find that it is best to start off with less expensive items and to invest in a superior model later on when they take their chosen sport or exercise more seriously.

Having the right clothing and equipment, however, can give you confidence.

Going out for a day's sailing will help you to stay fit and healthy. Out on the water you will have to protect your skin from strong sunshine and winds with a sunscreen or you may get very burnt indeed with the reflection off the water, even on hazy days.

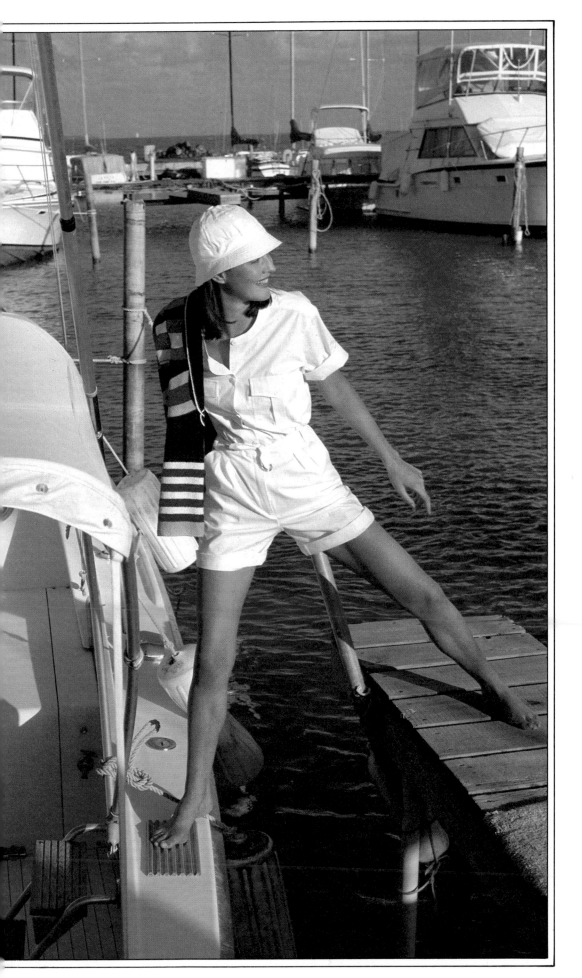

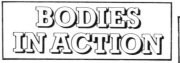
If you look the part, you are more likely to act the part too and to feel better doing it. A flattering tracksuit will help to make you feel like a real runner, and a fashionable, colourful leotard and tights will boost your self-confidence as a dancer. You will also feel more comfortable if you are dressed correctly. Most sports clothes are designed for comfort and ease of movement. Thus a short tennis skirt or shorts allows your legs to move more freely than tight hugging jeans. A leotard in a soft, stretchy fabric will not inhibit or restrict muscular or body movement when you go through your routine of stretching exercises. A loose, lightweight tracksuit will keep you warm in cold weather and allow the air to circulate freely around your body when you want to feel cool. Whatever you choose, it should always feel light and comfortable and it should wick perspiration away from your skin.

Well-made quality equipment can also help you to avoid injury. Every skiier knows that good skis with efficient bindings which release automatically in a tumble can save a broken limb. Likewise, good running shoes can make running easier and cushion your legs against the shock of pounding the ground 800 times per mile. Jogging in a pair of old tennis shoes puts enormous strain on your legs and every step you take will send shock waves through your skeleton and may jar your spine. There are many good models to choose from which are designed specifically for different surfaces and speeds. Thus there are studs for cross-country running, spikes for racing over mud, and lightweight shoes with wavy soles and good shock-absorption qualities for road running.

The right equipment can also improve your performance. For example, a light-weight racing bicycle with 10 speed gears is faster and easier to ride than a standard three-speed bike. A well strung tennis racket will have a larger area in its centre for hitting the ball true than a cheaper badly strung model. So don't skimp on your sporting gear if you want to take your exercise seriously and perform well. It is impossible to cover the whole range of sporting equipment here but we offer a guide to choosing the most common items:

Running shoes

Good shoes are important for any runner, new or experienced, as they take the shock of your every step. They are specially designed to make your running easier, more flowing and comfortable and to protect you from Achilles tendon, knee and leg injuries. The range of shoes is overwhelming — they come in so many colours, styles, materials and shapes. Your choice will depend on where you intend to run — on hard roads or across country. Grass and soft ground are better for beginners as they put less strain on your legs, so choose a waffle or studded sole for

Tracksuits are ideal for jogging and general leisure wear. Comfortable and non-restrictive to wear, they come in a wide range of flattering styles and colours. You can buy them in lightweight fabrics for summer, or warmer fleece-lined materials for winter wear. They are loose enough to allow maximum movement as you exercise.

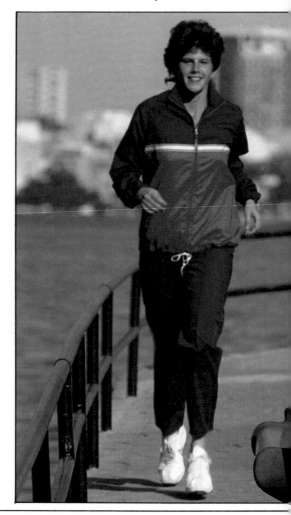

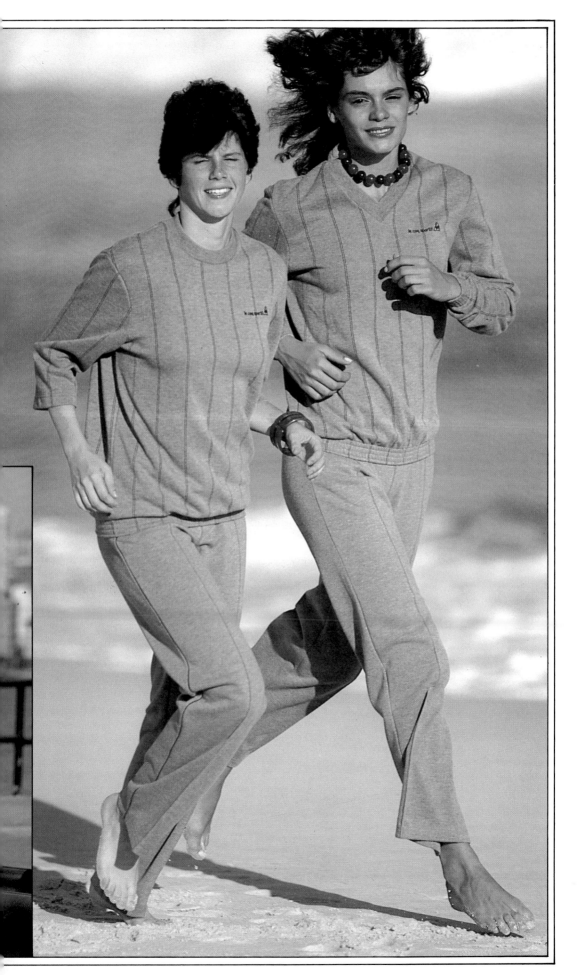

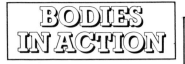

shock absorption and a better grip on uneven surfaces. The shoes should feel light, not heavy, and the heel tab should not be uncomfortable or irritate your Achilles tendon as you run. Try the shoes on in the store and walk around in them. Ask if you can jog about in front of the shop to test them out — they may feel different running on hard ground rather than walking on a soft padded carpet. Try different styles and remember that you will probably need a larger size than your normal shoe size for extra movement. Of course, running shoes are useful for other sports and exercise as well, including cycling, skipping and walking.

Tracksuits

These are excellent for running, cycling, working-out, playing tennis and other games in cold weather. They should feel light, loose and comfortable to wear, preferably with zip pockets for keeping keys and money safe. For cold or wet weather, choose ones which have hoods and a fleecy lining. Cheaper tracksuits which consist of cotton sweatshirts and pants are also suitable. They come in a wide range of colours and styles for the fashion-conscious among us.

Work-out wear

For working-out in a gym or exercise class, aerobic dancing, yoga or keep-fit, you can wear a loose, lightweight tracksuit, of course, but it is more fashionable and comfortable to dress in a leotard and footless ballet tights. Not only are they non-restricting to wear but they also make you more aware of your body and the muscular sensations you experience as you stretch and work-out. They come in a whole range of fashionable colours, patterns and styles although the more traditional ballet types are usually cheaper. Colourful leg warmers are fun to wear and keep your muscles warm while exercising, preventing stiffness.

Choosing the right sport

The exercise or sport you choose should feel right for you and satisfy your needs and natural abilities. First of all, you must decide what you want to get out of it. For

instance, do you want to develop overall fitness? Do you want to lose weight? Do you want to make new friends and have fun? Do you want an outdoor recreation or something you can practise at home? Your choice will also depend to some extent on where you live and the sports and leisure facilities that are available to you. Most towns now have a sports centre with a swimming pool, squash courts and gym. In addition, there may be an athletics track, a skating rink, tennis clubs, golf courses, exercise and dance studios. Some of these are reasonably priced, especially if they are run by your local authority, but the private clubs may be more expensive. Health and fitness clubs are now very popular and although the annual subscriptions may seem high they do offer many facilities and benefits which are really quite good value if calculated on a weekly basis.

Keep-fit and aerobic dance classes are booming everywhere, along with work-out, yoga, California stretch and jazz-aerobic sessions. Do not be nervous about attending these classes if they exist in your neighbourhood. Join up with a friend or go along on your own. You will meet many other like-minded people of all shapes, sizes and ages who have fun together, getting fit and healthy.

If you enjoy cycling or running, of course, you do not need any special facilities and you can exercise anywhere — in your local park, around the streets, on country lanes and paths. Special scenic cycle paths and jogging tracks are being slowly introduced in some places around the coast, along old canal towpaths or through the countryside where you can cycle or jog to your heart's content far away from traffic fumes and crowds. These are very popular in the States and are now being planned in Europe too. Special cycle lanes in towns and cities mean that you can cycle to work or the shops in relative safety.

If you live near a beach you have a wonderful opportunity to get really fit and

Wind-surfing is becoming a popular sport for many women. You can try it out on many lakes, reservoirs and harbours as well as at sea to develop strength and flexibility.

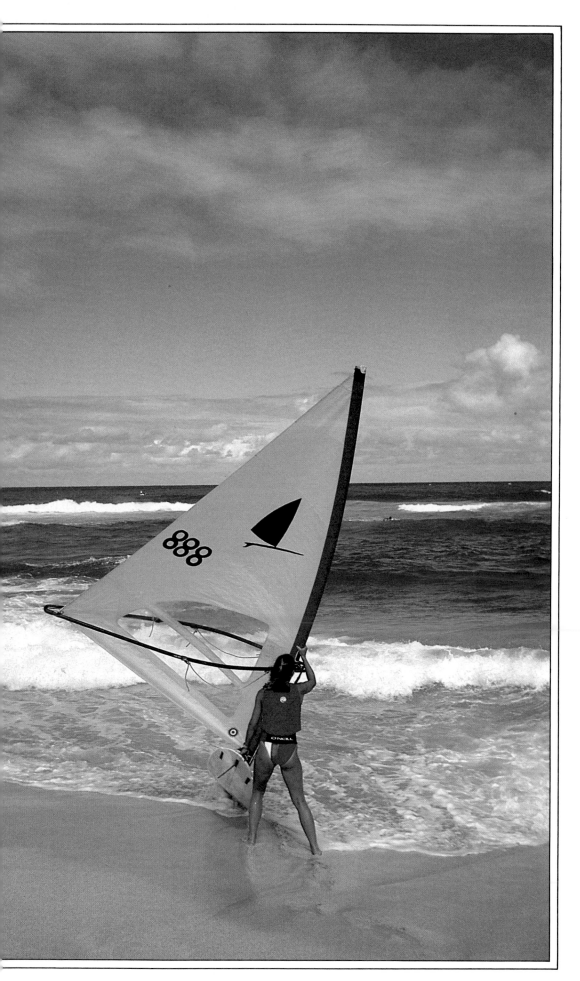

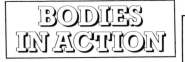
healthy. Swimming, surfing, water-skiing, wind-surfing and sailing are all healthy water-sports, and you can always jog along the beach and enjoy the sea-spray.

Only really vigorous aerobic sports burn up a lot of calories. Running hard can burn up over 800 calories per hour, jogging steadily can burn up 600, but golf accounts for only around 250 calories per hour. So if you want to exercise to lose weight or maintain a slim figure it is better to choose a really physical high-activity sport. Of course, not all aerobic sports will trim and condition your whole body — cycling and running are excellent for leg muscles, waist, hips and buttocks but not so effective for arms, so you may want to supplement these exercises with weights, tennis or squash. Look at the special tables to see how your sport rates in the calorie-burning and conditioning scales (page 57) and then on for a review of the most popular sports and physical activities and find out what they can do for you and how to get started if you are a complete beginner.

Running

The beauty of running is that you can do it at any age, anywhere and at any time. It's the ideal form of exercise — it's cheap, easy to master and you do not need any special sports facilities, just an open road, park or country lane where you can run. You can run all the year round in any weather and there is no better way to exercise aerobically. Running will strengthen your cardiovascular system so that your body processes oxygen more efficiently. It will make you slimmer too by burning up to 1000 calories per hour on a hard run, and depressing your appetite. In fact, you can expect to lose at least 5kg/10lb in your first year of running. And it can be as individual or as competitive as you wish it to be, as you race against other people or against yourself, setting your own targets to beat. More and more women are discovering the joys of running and fit it into their daily routine and work pattern. If you would like to try, here's how to get started.

If you haven't exercised regularly for a long time, are very overweight, smoke or drink heavily or have a family background of heart disease, it may be a good idea to have a medical check-up before you start. However, as running is used as a form of therapy for post-cardiac patients, it is unlikely that you will be unable to run provided that you take it slowly and build up your fitness gradually. The golden rule is train, don't strain. The best way to start is by alternating running with walking, building up the distance and your speed gradually. Start with running and walking for just 15 minutes and then gradually increase the time you are out. See chart on page 79 for a beginner's training schedule. Too many people try to run too fast initially before they become fit and supple, and usually get injured as a result as they put excessive strain on muscles which are unaccustomed to physical activity.

When to run

Only you can decide when it's best to fit running into your daily timetable. Whatever time you choose, whether it's first thing in the morning, at lunchtime or in the evening, make it a regular routine that you will not break. Never run immediately after eating — always allow an interval of at least two to three hours after eating solid foods. Don't rush your running either — allocate enough time to change, warm-up, go for your run, cool-down and shower afterwards (about one hour). Running should be relaxed and enjoyable.

How often?

Start by going out at least three times a week and as you get fitter and more supple you can go out more often. Do not run on consecutive days when you are starting out. Have a day's rest in between running days to allow your body time to recover. It may feel stiff at first but this feeling of discomfort will soon pass as you build up your general level of fitness. If the stiffness is very painful, however, and lasts for several days, then you have been over-doing it and have run either too fast or too far, so decrease your mileage and your speed next time you go out.

Running with a friend provides moral support and also encourages some healthy rivalry as together you strive towards new goals — to run further and faster.

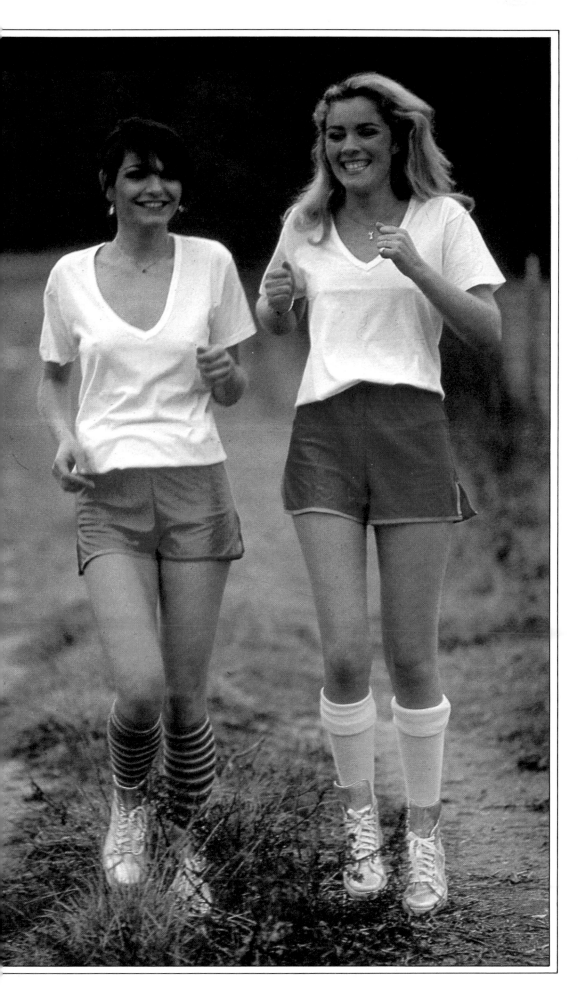

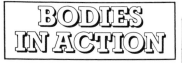
Where to run

Basically you can run anywhere — along city pavements, in your local park, around your neighbourhood, across country as long as you stick to common land and public footpaths, or on the beach. It's up to you. Try to run on grass most of the time as it is softer and less jarring to your spine than road-running. If you have to run a lot on roads, make sure that you wear good supportive shoes to cushion you against injury. Do not always choose the same running route as it may eventually become boring. Try a change of scenery occasionally by alternating several routes.

How far and how fast?

This depends on your personal fitness level, but to get aerobically fit you should run three to four times a week for 30 minutes. Choose a short route and start by running and walking it, gradually increasing the time you spend running and decreasing the periods of walking. When you can run all the way without any discomfort you can extend your distance and the pace at which you run. Your running speed will be affected by your physical condition, the weather, the terrain (whether it is flat or hilly) and the time of day. Running at the right speed, you should be able to hold a conversation without feeling winded or breathless. As the run progresses and you get your 'second wind', you will feel stronger and less laboured.

How to run

Running style is very important as developing a relaxed flowing style will make your running easier and more enjoyable. Never run stiffly or punch the air — instead, run tall, using your arms and shoulders to balance you, and let your body feel light and relaxed. There should be no feeling of tension or stiffness. Don't run daintily on your toes as many women tend to do — this puts too much strain on your leg muscles. Try to land heel-first to cushion your stride and develop a rocking action, landing on your heel, rocking forwards onto the ball of your foot and then pushing off again from the toes. Breathe through your mouth and take good gulps of air in a relaxed way in order to satisfy your body's oxygen needs and ensure a good flow to your muscles.

What to wear

Wear some loose comfortable clothing such as a sweatshirt or T-shirt and shorts, or a tracksuit. Your running shoes will be your most important and expensive item as they will provide essential support and cushioning and help you to avoid injury. Make sure that they fit comfortably with plenty of room between your big toe and

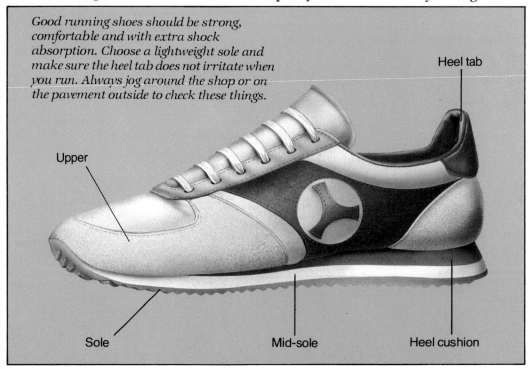

Good running shoes should be strong, comfortable and with extra shock absorption. Choose a lightweight sole and make sure the heel tab does not irritate when you run. Always jog around the shop or on the pavement outside to check these things.

Heel tab

Upper

Sole

Mid-sole

Heel cushion

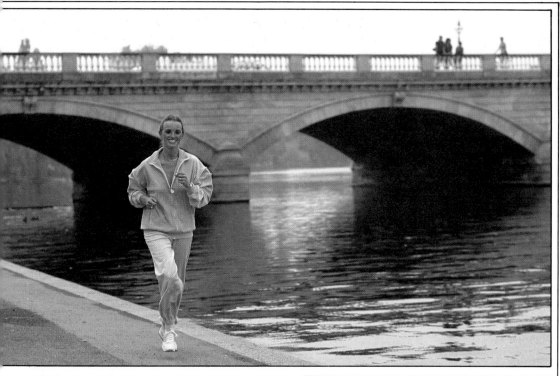

The beauty of running is that you can run anywhere at any time of day you like.

the end of the shoe. Choose a flat, wavy sole for roadwork; a studded or waffle sole for running across country and uneven ground. Wrap up warmly in cold weather to prevent catching a chill, and be sure to wear reflective armbands and light clothing if you run at night after dark.

Warming up and cooling down

It is vital to warm-up and stretch out your muscles before you set out for a run. This will ease and relax tense muscles, and prevent post-run stiffness. Stretching improves flexibility and increases mobility so that the risk of injury is less. Warming-up will raise your pulse rate and prepare you for the act of running itself. For some suggestions, see the illustrations on page... Cooling-down and stretching after a run relaxes the muscles and allows your pulse rate to return to normal. Do not skimp on these routines, make them a regular part of your training and you will feel fitter, more relaxed and supple.

Running schedule

This programme was specially designed by John Hanscomb, an experienced runner who trains beginners who want to compete in the London Marathon. He thinks that new runners often find it easier to follow a specially designed running programme than to devise their own. Here are his suggestions for building up gradually:

Training programme

Weeks 1,2,3,4
Run/walk for 15 minutes, 3 times a week until you can run 15 minutes non-stop.

Weeks 5,6,7,8
Weekdays: run/walk for 20 minutes, 3 times a week.
Weekends: run/walk for 30 minutes on Saturday *or* Sunday.
Keep this up until you can run non-stop for the times given above.

Weeks 9,10
Sunday: very slow run for 45 minutes, perhaps with occasional walk.
Monday: steady run for 20 minutes.
Tuesday: steady run for 30 minutes.
Wednesday: rest.
Thursday: run for 15-20 minutes at a brisk pace.
Friday: steady run for 20 minutes
Saturday: rest.

Weeks 11,12
Sunday: slow run for 45 minutes without walking.
Monday: steady run for 20 minutes.
Tuesday: steady run for 30 minutes.
Wednesday: steady run for 20 minutes.
Thursday: hard run for 15-20 minutes.
Friday: rest.
Saturday: steady run for 20-25 minutes.

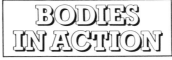

Water-sports

Most water-sports offer a marvellous and enjoyable way to get fit, especially if you live by the sea or near a large lake where you can sail, water-ski or wind-surf. However, swimming, which is a cheap and most effective form of aerobic exercise, can be practised in your local pool and will give your body one of the best all-over work-outs it can get.

Swimming

If you cannot swim already, then swimming lessons from experienced instructors are available at most swimming baths and pools. It does not take long to learn as the water supports you as you move along. It is a wonderful way of toning up your body if practised regularly — at least three times a week — and is particularly suitable for people with weight, muscular and back problems. It firms and strengthens the muscles in your lower and upper back, reshaping and steamlining your whole body. And, of course, the harder and faster you swim, the more calories you use even though the support of the water and the buoyant nature of your body makes the effort seem less than it really is. Unlike many forms of exercise, there is little risk of getting injured as your body is practically weightless in the water and you do not strain it so much as, say, in running or a game of tennis or squash.

To get long lasting effects and aerobic conditioning you must swim regularly, starting perhaps with 15 minutes' non-stop swimming backwards and forwards along the length of the pool, and gradually working up to 30 minutes or more. Try to choose a time of day when the pool is not too crowded so that you can swim continuously without stopping. Stop for a rest when you begin to feel tired but this will become less frequent as your level of fitness improves. You can wear goggles to protect your eyes if the chlorine irritates them. If you are fortunate enough to live close to the sea, then summer swimming along the coast is even more fun and less monotonous. Your body will soon warm up as it gets accustomed to the water temperature and you expend more energy. Always swim in a safe place where

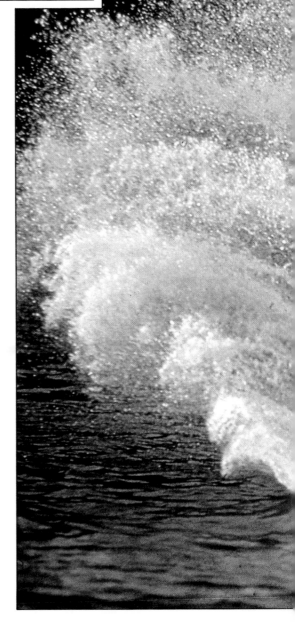

there are no dangerous currents and come ashore if the danger flags are raised on the beach. Also, beware of going out too far in case of cramp — it may be a long swim back.

Surfing

Although women surfers were rare until a few years ago, they are now becoming more common on the beaches of the United States, Australia, Britain and Europe. Riding the surf and the huge white breakers as they roll in towards the shore is exhilarating and fun. It is also a good way of staying fit and healthy. Although it will not build up overall fitness, surfing can help you to develop strong arm and

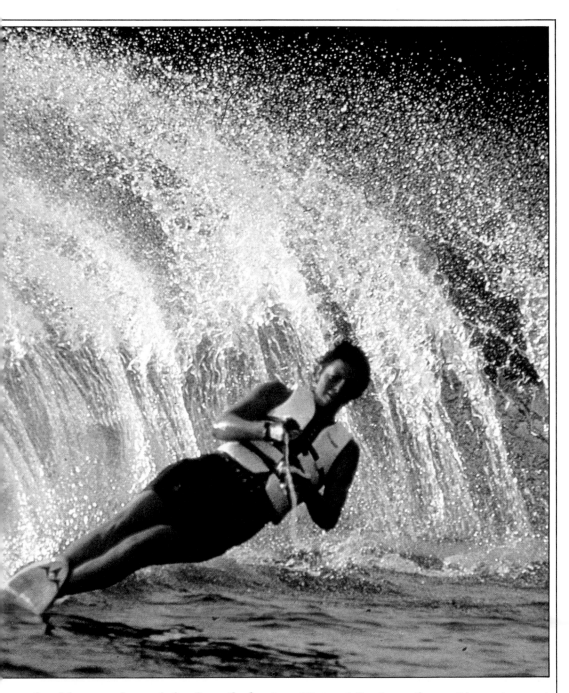

shoulder muscles and also firms the bust. You should supplement it by running, swimming or some other form of aerobic exercise. All you need is a super light-weight surfboard which is narrow and streamlined with a stabilising fin at the back. You do not even have to venture out of your depth to surf successfully. However, you *do* need good surf.

You have to paddle the board out to a point where the waves are rising and then wait until you catch a big wave. You rise up from a crouch into a standing position on top of the board as the wave swells beneath you. The aim is to ride the wave into the shore, using your rear foot to navigate the board. Large breakers may

Water-skiing is another exciting water sport which will make your body firmer, leaner and stronger too. You need to be a good swimmer in case you take a tumble. You can ski alone or even in formation behind a fast motorboat which skims across the surface of the water at about 20 miles per hour.

be as high as four metres so you need a good sense of balance and a flexible, and supple body to succeed.

Surfing originated in Hawaii, which probably has the best breakers in the world, but it is now popular everywhere, especially in California and Australia where the climate is warm. In colder European countries, you will probably need to wear a wetsuit!

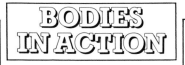
Wind-surfing

Enthusiasts would claim that this sport is even more exciting and demanding than surfing as you have to ride the wind as well as the waves. It started as a combination of sailing, skiing and surfing in California in the 1960s, and because it is a cheap alternative to sailing and an enjoyable way of getting fit, it soon spread to Europe and Australia. A good way of conditioning your body, it can be as difficult and as challenging as you care to make it, as you can choose your own speed and decide whether you wish to venture out on a warm day to ride smoother water in light winds, or to wait for a choppy sea and a bumpy ride!

The idea is to move in tune with the wind and waves and gradually develop your flexibility and technique until you capsize only rarely. You do not have to be tall and strong as much as fit and really supple to succeed at this sport. To develop cardiovascular fitness and endurance, it is a good idea to supplement your wind-surfing with an aerobic exercise. You will have to practise and persevere until you master the art but it will get easier as your muscle tone improves and you feel fitter.

Many established schools exist to teach you how to wind-surf, or board-sail as it is sometimes called. You will have to expect a lot of duckings at first but as you become more experienced these will probably become less. On all but the warmest summer days you will probably need to wear a wetsuit, possibly with a light windproof jacket over the top. You can practise on many lakes, rivers and reservoirs as well as at sea. Beginners must take care in open water and check the weather forecast before setting out, as only very experienced sailors should attempt to wind-surf in strong offshore winds. Try to sail in company if possible so that help is available if you need it, and always tell someone where you are going and at what time you expect to return so that they can alert the rescue authorities if necessary. Don't be put off by this advice as it is common sense and quite normal for anyone going out sailing at sea. Obviously it is safer to learn on an inland waterway, lake, estuary or harbour where help is nearby if you need it. Wind-surfing is restricted in some areas so check that it is indeed permissible before you leave shore.

Sailing

Exhilarating and great fun, sailing is a marvellous way of getting out into the open air and unwinding. You experience a sense of totality and peacefulness when you are out on the ocean, maybe miles from land with just the great expanse of sea and sky around you as far as you can see. It is doubtful that sailing alone will get you fit unless you sail single-handed in strong seas, which is demanding and potentially dangerous, but you can burn up a lot of calories on a blustery day when you are working hard changing sails and tacking with the wind. On

Surfing (below) and underwater diving (right) are strictly for the more adventurous. You will need to get kitted out with the right equipment before you venture above or below the waves! It is important to have expert instruction in diving to learn all about the safety aspects and using equipment.

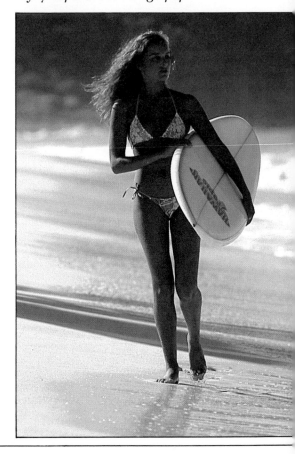

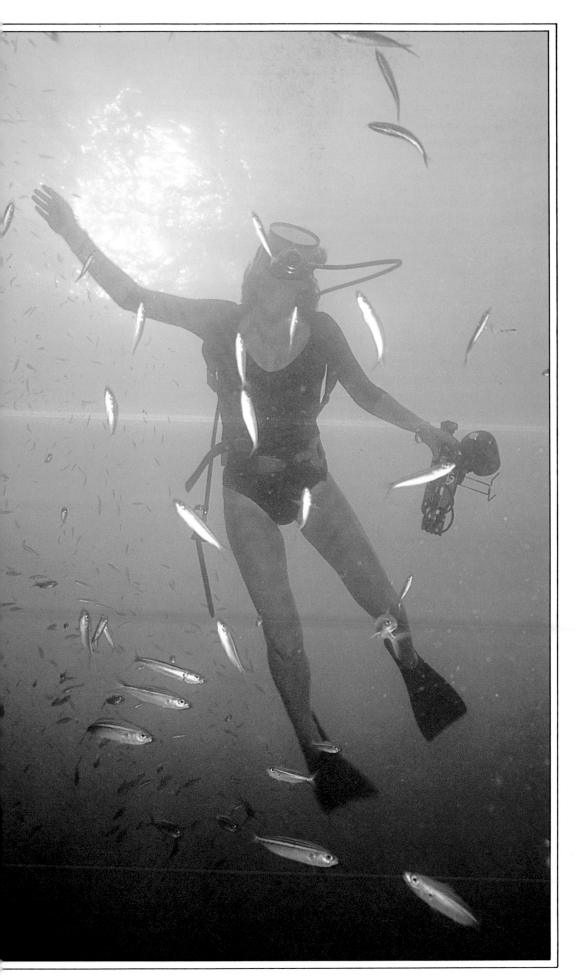

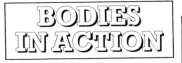

calmer warmer days, it is tempting to stretch out on the deck in the sun and let others do the work, keeping physical activity down to a minimum.

Whatever type and size of boat you sail, it is important to learn the basics before you leave the harbour for the first time. For example, there is a strict code of conduct for safety at sea which has to be observed by all boats, including right of way, laws of the sea etc. You will need to learn how to control, sail and navigate a small boat, how to use a radio, put up sails, change course and many other things. There are several ways of learning — by crewing for friends, by answering advertisements for crew in yachting magazines, or by enrolling for special lessons from qualified instructors. Many sailing courses are held on inland reservoirs and lakes as well as at coastal resorts.

On deck, always wear rubber, canvas or rope-soled shoes to protect the decks against marks and damage and also for safety as they will provide better gripping when the boat starts to list. Even on warm days, it is a good idea to take some weatherproofs with you as there can be a bracing breeze out at sea and conditions can change very quickly with little warning. Sailing can be an expensive business if you plan to have your own boat as mooring fees can be high in harbours and marinas and general maintenance can be costly too, but if you sail regularly and enjoy it, it is well worth the expense.

Cycling

Burning up about 660 calories per hour, cycling ranks among the best cardio-respiratory exercises. Not only is it a cheap and practical way to travel but it is also an enjoyable way to get fit and slim, as it strengthens your heart as well as your muscles, improves circulation and increases your lung power. It is a great way to get about and see the countryside, or just to go from A to B in busy city traffic. To benefit aerobically from cycling, you will have to go out at least three times a week, gradually building up to five or six sessions. If you cycle to work or the shops every day you will soon start to feel stronger

and fitter, but going out for a long distance cycle just once a week is more likely to do you harm than good as you may subject your body to excessive strain. Like running or any other aerobic exercise, cycling must be practised regularly if is to do you any good. As you become more proficient you will be able to cover greater distances faster and more comfortably. However, you might feel unfit or breathless on the first few occasions that you go out, and will need some recovery time. Start off by cycling on alternate days for about 30 minutes, and then build up the time you spend out on your bike to about one hour with a longer cycle at weekends. It is a good sport for all the family to share and you can always make it a day out by packing a picnic lunch into your cycle bags or baskets.

Road safety

As a cyclist you may be vulnerable on busy roads so it is just as well to know and observe the rules of the road. Always ride in single file, and *not* two abreast so that it is difficult for cars to pass you. Try to anticipate the actions of motorists and make your intentions clear to them also, remembering to give handsignals when turning. In busy traffic, cycle in a straight line staying well to the side of the road. Do not be tempted to weave your way through the traffic jams. At busy intersections and roundabouts it is sometimes better and safer to dismount and wheel your bike across rather than cut your way through moving lanes of traffic.

If you cycle after dusk, make sure that your lights work efficiently. As an added precaution wear a white jacket with reflective strips to show up in car head-lights. Be on the look-out for car doors opening in front of you when motorists are parked on the kerb. Keep your bike in good running order by checking it over regularly and keep a basic tool kit in your saddle bag for emergencies. You can go to special classes to learn how to maintain your bike in good running order, repair punctures and replace brake cables and other simple jobs.

Opposite: A racing bike with drop handle bars and 10-speed gears will enable you to cycle much faster than a 3-speed model.

Before you set out on a long cycle ride, check the following:

1 That you have a pump and repair kit in case of punctures.

2 That your brakes work efficiently.

3 That the air pressure in the tyres is correct.

4 That all the nuts and bolts are tight.

5 That the wheels are properly aligned.

6 That the handlebars are tight.

7 That the chain is properly adjusted and lubricated with oil, as are all other moving parts.

8 That the frame is straight and not warped.

9 That the seat is adjusted to its proper height.

10 That the lights and bell are working properly.

11 That you have a padlock to secure your bike should you leave it in front of the shops or any other public place. Remember that cycles are the easiest thing in the world to steal and they are difficult to trace. However, you can have the serial number engraved on the frame which makes the job of the police easier if your bike is stolen.

Choosing a bike

When it comes to buying a bike, there are many different styles and frame sizes to choose from — racing bikes, fold-away bikes, small-wheeled 'shoppers', large touring bikes — the list is endless. First of all, analyse your reasons for owning a bike — do you want it for pottering around your neighbourhood, for getting super-fit and racing, or for cycle tours? A normal three-speed gear model is suitable for cycling short distances, but a lightweight racing bike with five- or 10-speed gears would be better for covering rough ground or touring.

To discover which size is best for you, sit astride some different models with both feet placed flat on the ground. On a bike with a horizontal bar, there should be a clearance of 4cm/1½in between the bar and the top of your legs. Then adjust the seat height until you can sit on the saddle and *just* reach the ground with your feet either side, or until your leg on

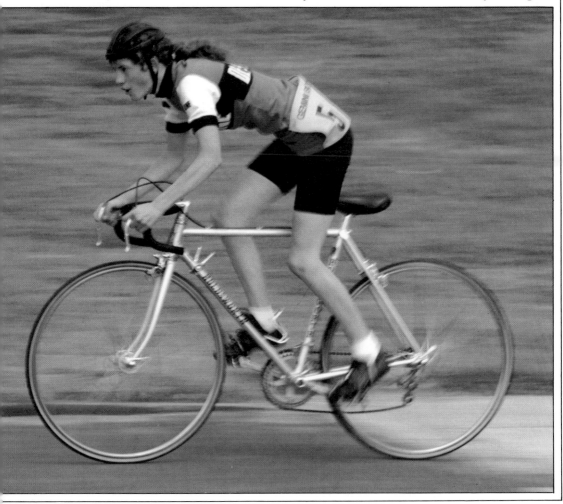

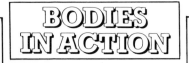

the downstroke pedal is almost fully extended. If the seat is too high you will not be able to reach the pedal — too low and you will not use your leg muscles properly and will be vulnerable to cramp.

Try out several sizes until you discover the best 'fit' for you. The small-wheeled bicycles are easy to store and are very manoeuvrable in city traffic. However, they have a low centre of gravity and you have to pedal harder than on a larger-wheeled model, which gives you an easier ride. The large wheels even out rough surfaces so· that they feel smoother and less bumpy.

The great outdoors

Walking, hiking, rock climbing, canoeing, mountaineering and many other outdoor sports and activities can help keep you fit and active and may provide a challenge in your life. Some people thrive on dangerous activities where they need to bring their special skills and personal qualities into play. Although walking is basic to everyone, you will need to go on a special course if you are thinking of taking up climbing or canoeing, say, for the first time. Demanding, exhilarating and immense fun, all these sports require courage and determination and will help you to get to know yourself and your limitations and to increase your self-confidence. Traditionally regarded as masculine activities, many women are now taking them up and succeeding where once they would not have dared to venture for fear of being ridiculed by men.

Even walking, perhaps the most underrated of all physical activities, can make you fit and healthy and help you to discover the countryside. Going out for long walks at weekends is exhilarating and relaxing —a way to get away from it all and the pressures and strains of your everyday life as you discover new sights, routes and beautiful places. You can build walking into your daily routine too, so that you walk to work or the shops instead of bussing or taking the car. Walk upstairs in preference to taking the elevator. Go for a walk in your lunch-hour instead of remaining at your desk. As long as you have low-heeled comfortable shoes, you can walk anywhere at any time. Walk

briskly and with a natural rhythm for three or four miles a day and you will soon feel fitter and more supple.

Walking a golf course is another way of staying fit and active, although you would have to play for at least five hours every day to get really fit. However, it is relaxing and fun and gets you outside. As it is foremost a game of technique you will need some expert tuition before you hit your local golf course. So don't rush out and buy an expensive set of clubs — have some lessons first and practise with some cheap second-hand equipment on your local municipal or public course before you join a club. Many golf clubs now recruit women members and women's golf is a fast- growing sport.

When the summer comes, many people make a dash for the tennis courts. There are no age limits as many people who only discover the game in their thirties or forties can testify. As long as you are reasonably supple and mobile you are never too old to play. If you haven't played since your schooldays, you should take a refresher course on service, footwork and basic strokes. Injuries usually occur when you do not play properly and over-strain muscles unused to strenuous physical activity. Once you know the basics, you must practise them until they become second-nature and you build up the speed and technique to partner more accomplished players.

You will need a racket, either in wood, aluminium, steel or fibreglass. Try holding different models in the shop and test them for weight and size — you should be able to touch the top of your third finger with your thumb when you grip the handle firmly. As a beginner, an inexpensive racket strung with nylon is probably most suitable, but as you gain experience and evelop a greater commitment to the game, you can invest in a gut-strung more expensive model. However, don't cheat on tennis shoes — they have to absorb the shock of a lot of movement on a hard court and should be comfortable.

Tennis is an exciting game, whether it is played by amateurs or by top players such as Hannah Mandalikova — shown here in action at Wimbledon, England.

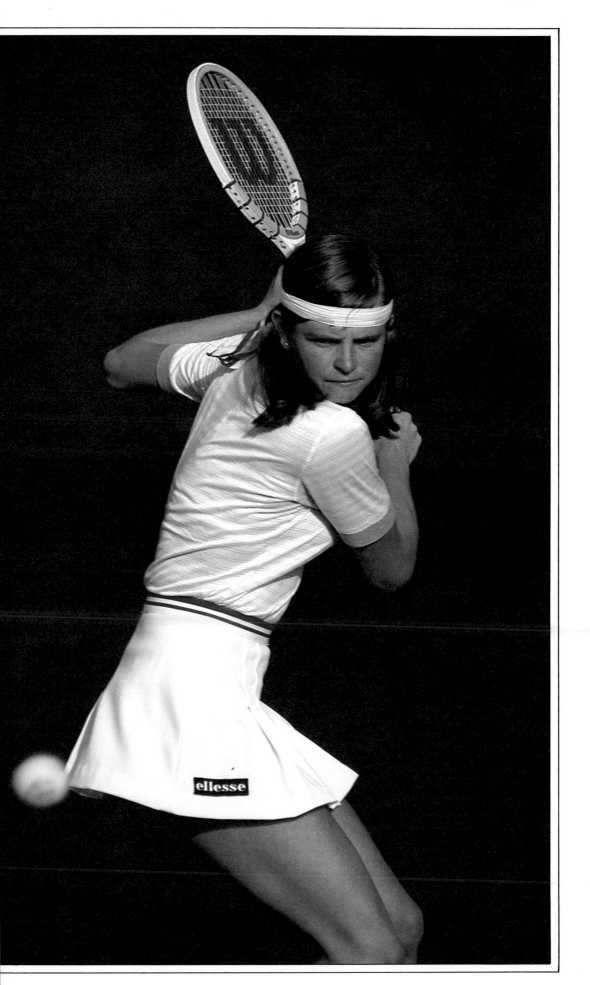

Jackie Genova

For Jackie Genova, exercise and aerobics star of British television, exercise is "as natural as cleaning my teeth." Jackie works out every day, either at her own exercise studio or in front of the cameras in her regular slot on TV-AM's breakfast show. A top model in her native Sydney, she went to study aerobic exercise under Jane Fonda herself in California.

"All my life I've exercised and wanted to keep fit. I've always worked-out in some way or another because I knew that it was the best way to keep my weight down. At home in Australia, I used to jog on the beach at 6.30 every morning. When I came to London I ran in Hyde Park most days but it meant that I had to get up very early to take classes or appear on TV."

Jackie certainly is busy — opening up another studio in London's West End and launching her book *Work that body*.

She thinks that the fitness and exercise boom is here to stay once people discover the benefits of being fit. "Most people don't know their own bodies but they're interested and want to learn. They also want to be convinced that keeping fit is good for them. After a while they rely on exercise for getting the best out of life."

She also thinks that if you do too much exercise it can be counter-productive and even ageing for some women. "I used to do five or six hours every day but now I do less. For most people, just four times a week is enough to keep their bodies feeling great and fit. After a work-out you feel terrific and as though you've achieved something. I like it when it's really hard. I would never exercise without warming-up first. It really makes you feel better, especially if you're tired, and then I go into 12 minutes of jogging or aerobics."

Jackie always works-out to music. "It pumps up adrenalin in the body and makes you work harder, especially if you like the record! Sometimes I wear ankle or leg weights too. When you exercise you speed up your metabolism, repair muscle fibres that are naturally destroyed and keep your weight down."

After years of dieting, Jackie discovered that regular exercise and good nutrition are the best ways of staying slim. "For years I wouldn't dream of looking at bread and the things my body needed. I went through a very destructive phase once when I ate practically no fibre. Now I eat more healthily. I have two slices of toast and muesli for breakfast. I have a salad or sandwich at lunchtime, and if I'm starving in the evening I eat liver and spinach."

"When most people start exercising they change their eating habits naturally and eat the food that's good for them. The best change in me was when I stopped drinking. I felt a real glow inside. I didn't have a drink for eight months although now I have one occasionally. I drink mineral water most of the time. I used to

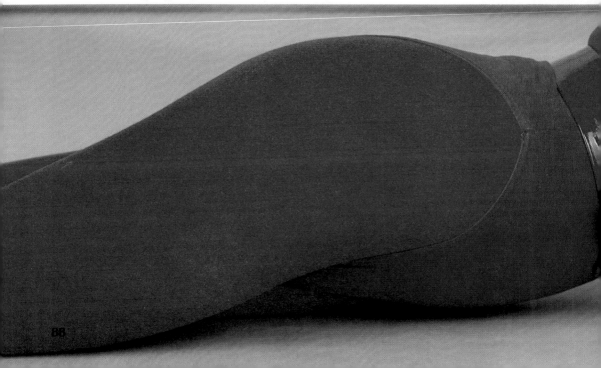

smoke too but gave that up about 18 months ago. Exercise was a wonderful help as it made the cigarettes taste awful. I only wish I'd done all these things 10 years ago.''

You have to be really fit and supple to stretch as far as Jackie Genova but with regular practice, you too can be this mobile and flexible. Working-out is an effective and really enjoyable way of toning up your body and trimming away any areas of flab. You can lose literally inches off your waistline, stomach, hips and thighs in a few weeks.

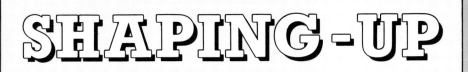

SHAPING-UP

Now that you know about sport and the different types of exercise, you can concentrate on shaping up any areas of your body which are crying out for special attention. Here is the complete work-out to do at home for strengthening your body and making it more flexible and supple all over. And there is also a short section on working out with weights to stay slim and firm. Whichever method you prefer, they are both great ways of keeping your figure trim and youthful, and practised regularly, say, three or four times a week, it will only be a matter of weeks before you see some positive results and all your hard work is rewarded. Moreover, shaping up is fun and as you get fitter you will really enjoy your work-out or weight-training sessions, whether you do it on your own at home or in your local gym or exercise studio with other enthusiasts.

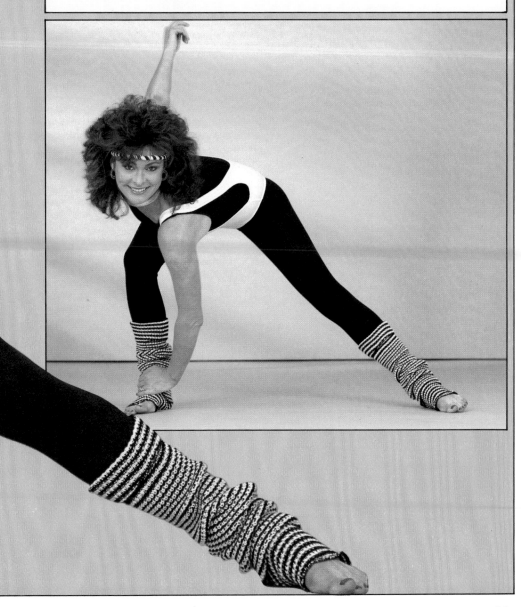

Your own work-out programme

This special work-out programme in easy-to-follow step-by-step pictures was devised by the experts at Holmes Place Health Club in London and is performed overleaf by instructor Cheryl Holmes. The exercises are suitable for beginners and are perfectly safe if you follow the instructions carefully and do them correctly. Study the pictures and familiarise yourself with the exercises shown. Practise them until you can perform them smoothly in the correct sequence without referring back to the book.

The work-out is geared to working every area of your body for all-over conditioning and toning — your arms, shoulders, waist, stomach, back, hips, legs and buttocks. Practised regularly, it will improve your muscle tone, strengthen your heart and cardiovascular endurance, improve your circulation, and make you slimmer and fitter. For maximum benefit you should work-out at least three times a week for roughly 30 minutes per session. It will be difficult at first and you will sweat a lot but it will get easier, and afterwards you will feel refreshed and full of energy.

As you become more advanced, you can try out variations on the exercises given, stretching further and harder; and increase your warm-up and aerobics time and the number of repetitions of each exercise. To work-out sucessfully at home takes self-discipline and dedication

if it is to become a regular commitment. Choose a regular time, and put it aside for your work-out.

You may prefer to work-out in a class under the eye of a qualified instructor with other people. If so, use this work-out programme to supplement your classes or as a filler if you miss a class. If you like working-out to music, choose a record with a strong beat — most disco music is suitable. Make sure that you sustain your concentration on the work-out itself and don't get carried away by the music. Choose a place where you can be alone and uninterrupted. There should be enough room to jump up and swing your arms to the sides and above your head, and to stretch out in all directions for floorwork. Make sure that you have a mat, towel or rug ready for when you start the floor exercises.

Work evenly on both sides of the body — you may unknowingly be working-out harder on one side than on the other and this will produce very uneven results. Listen to what your body is telling you and respect it. Don't push it too hard until you are fit and can take the extra strain. Go for quality — not quantity. It is better to perform a few exercises really well than to try and do more and skimp on them or to do them badly.

Do the exercises in the sequence given and never cheat or miss out the warm-up and warm-down — these are important parts of the total programme. Don't be disappointed if you don't get instantly fit and slim — it takes time, practice and patience to build up endurance, strength and stamina and to 'work' those excess inches off your waist, hips and thighs.Have a warm shower or bath to relax and ease out muscles and limbs. As you become more proficient and your personal level of fitness increases, the stiffness will pass.

Lastly, while you work-out it is vitally important to breathe correctly — not small shallow gasps but deep breaths right from your abdomen. Breathe in through your nose and out through your mouth. Keep it regular and deep to maintain a steady flow of oxygen to your muscles.

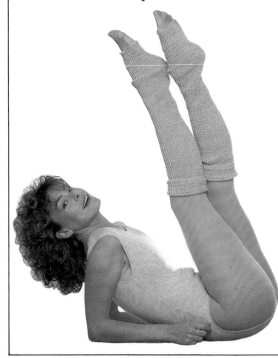

When working-out, it is a good idea to wear leg-warmers like Jackie does to keep muscles warm and prevent stiffness and soreness afterwards.

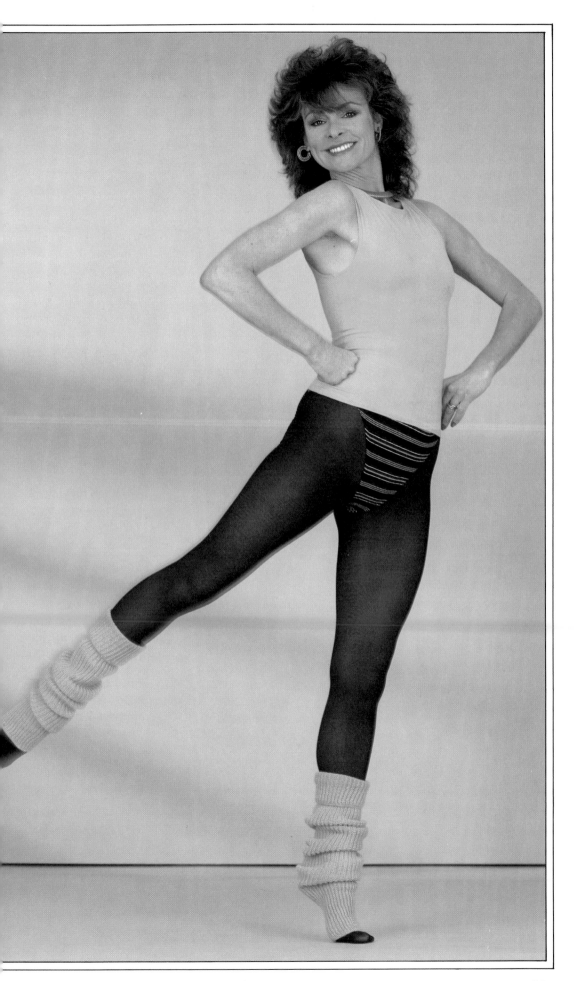

Warm-up

At the start of the work-out always warm-up to improve blood circulation to the muscles, increase your pulse rate, and stretch out muscles. This will reduce the risk of injury and get you in the right mood and condition for the work-out proper.

Neck stretches and head rolls

1 *Stand with your feet hip distance apart, arms by your sides and stomach and buttocks pulled in tightly. Now stretch your neck to the left and hold for a count of 2.*

2 *Stretch your neck to the right and hold for a count of 2. Repeat 8 times on each side. Now roll your head to the left for 2 counts, back for another 2 counts, to the right for 2 counts and then forwards. Now reverse and repeat. Do 2 more rolls to each side. If you are performing the exercise correctly you should feel the pull in your neck.*

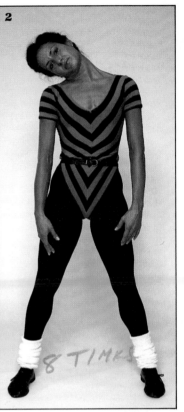

Shoulder circles

1 *Stand with your feet a little more than shoulder distance apart. Lift your right shoulder up towards your right ear and move it backwards in a circular movement, lowering it and raising it again. Repeat 8 times. Now reverse and circle it forwards 8 times.*

2 *Repeat this exercise 8 times backwards with your left shoulder, and then 8 times forwards with your left shoulder. This exercise will help you to loosen up.*

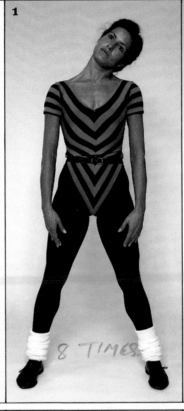

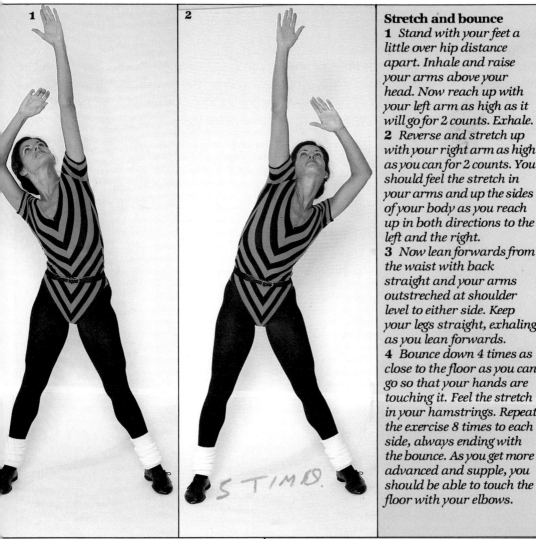

1

2

5 TIMES.

Stretch and bounce
1 *Stand with your feet a little over hip distance apart. Inhale and raise your arms above your head. Now reach up with your left arm as high as it will go for 2 counts. Exhale.*
2 *Reverse and stretch up with your right arm as high as you can for 2 counts. You should feel the stretch in your arms and up the sides of your body as you reach up in both directions to the left and the right.*
3 *Now lean forwards from the waist with back straight and your arms outstreched at shoulder level to either side. Keep your legs straight, exhaling as you lean forwards.*
4 *Bounce down 4 times as close to the floor as you can go so that your hands are touching it. Feel the stretch in your hamstrings. Repeat the exercise 8 times to each side, always ending with the bounce. As you get more advanced and supple, you should be able to touch the floor with your elbows.*

3

4

8 TIMES

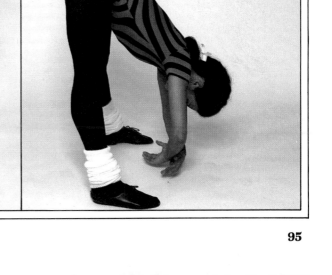

Aerobics

The aerobic part of the work-out will raise your pulse rate higher and get you well and truly warmed up for the coming exercises. Try to breathe evenly and deeply all the time and slow down and walk on the spot if you become breathless or dizzy. The important thing is to get your blood carrying more oxygen to your muscles.

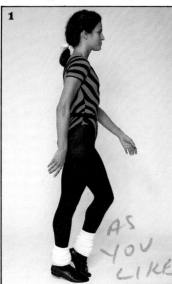

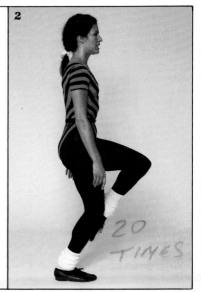

1 Foot rolling
Start off gently with foot rolling to get your upper and lower body moving. Just walk on the spot, rolling on the balls of your feet, as many times as you like until you feel really warmed-up.

2 Jogging in place
Jog on the spot for 20 counts, landing on your toes and then touching down with your heels. Now raise your knees higher and jog for 20 counts with raised knees. Keep on breathing deeply.

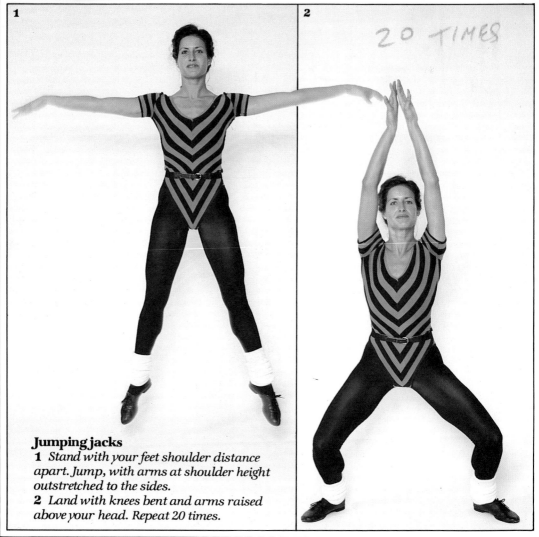

Jumping jacks
1 *Stand with your feet shoulder distance apart. Jump, with arms at shoulder height outstretched to the sides.*
2 *Land with knees bent and arms raised above your head. Repeat 20 times.*

Boxing twist
Stand with feet shoulder distance apart. Twist to the left, punching with left arm outstretched and right arm bent close to body. Reverse and repeat 15 times.

15 TIMES.

Skipping
Use a real or an imaginary skipping rope for this exercise. Breathe deeply and regularly, jumping just high enough to clear the rope and looking straight ahead — not at the rope. Gradually build up the rhythm. Start off with 40 skips forwards, and as you get more advanced, increase the repetitions and try skipping backwards as well. Wear shoes for extra shock absorption.

40 TIMES.

1

2

20 TIMES

Calf stretch
1 Stand with your right leg stretched back behind you, only the toes on the ground, and left leg bent in front of you, with your whole foot flat on the ground.
2 Now lower the heel of your right leg slowly to the floor. Bounce gently up and down for 20 counts so that you feel the stretch in your calf muscles on the downwards bounce. Reverse and repeat with the left leg for 20 counts.

Arms and shoulders

These exercises will help strengthen your arm, shoulder and chest muscles, making them more supple and flexible. Remember to keep breathing steadily and easily throughout, and really work those arms hard to achieve positive results.

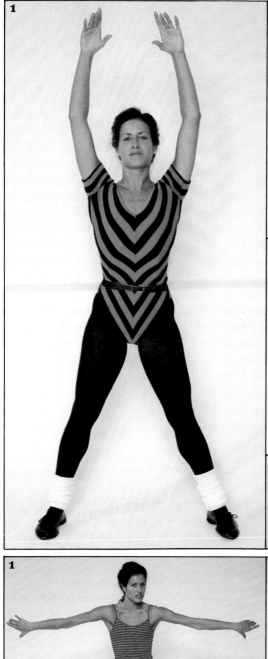

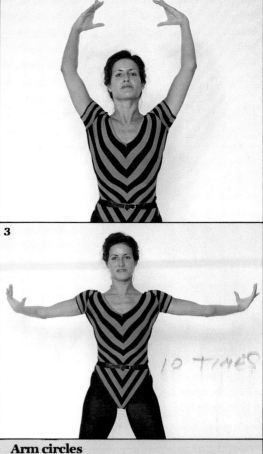

10 TIMES

Arm circles

1 *Stand with your feet a little over hip distance apart, arms raised above head.*
2 *Bend your arms slightly and circle them forwards with wrists flexed for 10 counts.*
3 *Circle them backwards for 10 counts.*

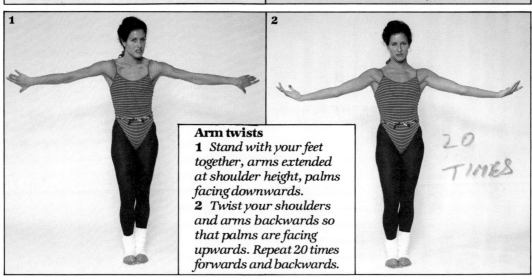

Arm twists

1 *Stand with your feet together, arms extended at shoulder height, palms facing downwards.*
2 *Twist your shoulders and arms backwards so that palms are facing upwards. Repeat 20 times forwards and backwards.*

20 TIMES

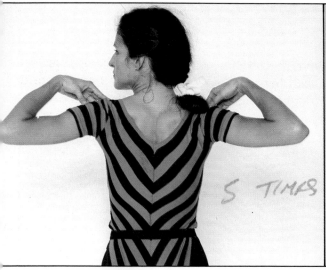

S TIMES

◄ Pectoral stretch
Stand with your feet shoulder distance apart, arms at shoulder height, elbows bent with hands resting on shoulders. Keeping your shoulders back, stretch backwards for 2 counts, and then forwards for 2 counts. Repeat 5 times.

Arm scissors
1 *Stand with your feet shoulder distance apart, arms behind your back, and hands crossed.*
2 *Now scissor your arms backwards and forwards 20 times, keeping them extended behind your back.*
▼

1
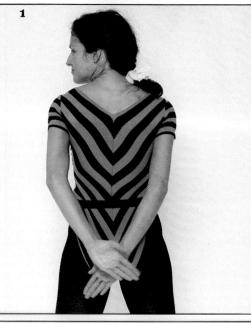

2
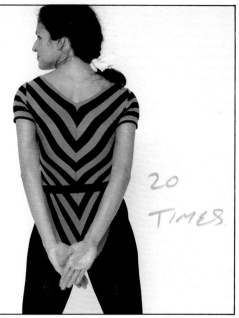

20 TIMES.

1
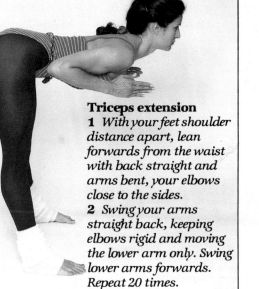

Triceps extension
1 *With your feet shoulder distance apart, lean forwards from the waist with back straight and arms bent, your elbows close to the sides.*
2 *Swing your arms straight back, keeping elbows rigid and moving the lower arm only. Swing lower arms forwards. Repeat 20 times.*

2
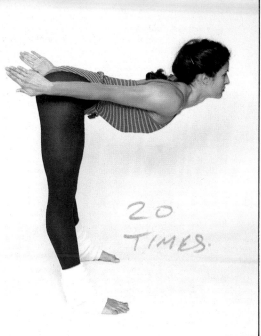

20 TIMES.

Waists

These waist exercises will help strengthen the muscles in this area and reduce your waistline, making it trimmer and firmer. They are also good for toning up and strengthening the lower back muscles, making you less prone to back ache.

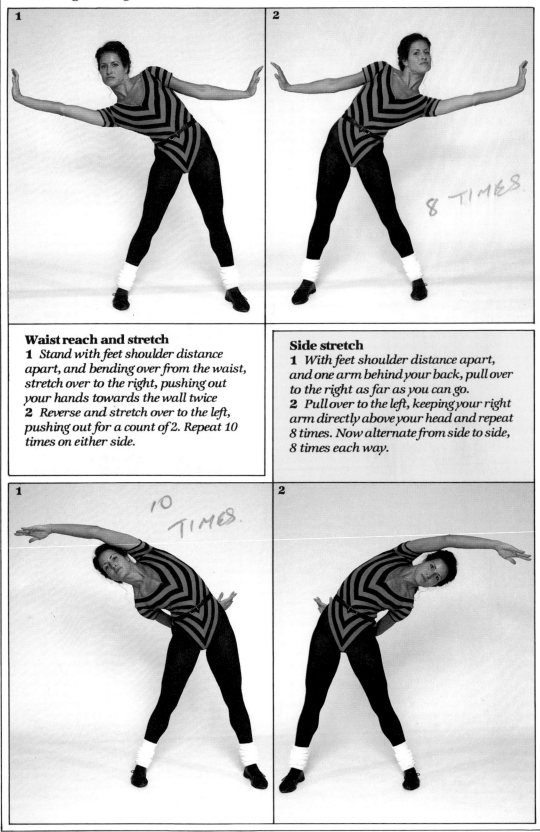

Waist reach and stretch
1 *Stand with feet shoulder distance apart, and bending over from the waist, stretch over to the right, pushing out your hands towards the wall twice*
2 *Reverse and stretch over to the left, pushing out for a count of 2. Repeat 10 times on either side.*

Side stretch
1 *With feet shoulder distance apart, and one arm behind your back, pull over to the right as far as you can go.*
2 *Pull over to the left, keeping your right arm directly above your head and repeat 8 times. Now alternate from side to side, 8 times each way.*

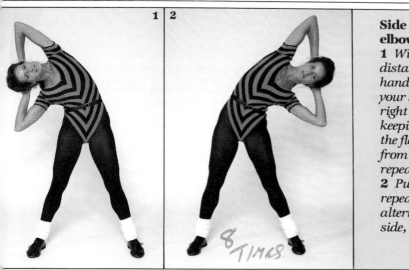

Side stretch with elbows

1 *With feet shoulder distance apart, and both hands clasped behind your head, pull over to the right as far as you can go, keeping your feet flat on the floor and bending from the waist only. Now repeat 8 times.*

2 *Pull over to the left and repeat 8 times. Now alternate from side to side, 8 times each way*

8 TIMES

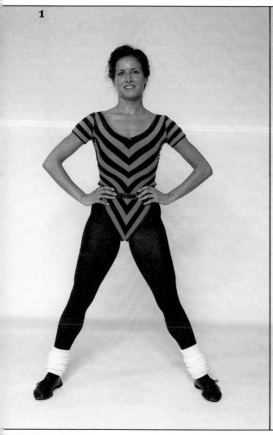

8 TIMES

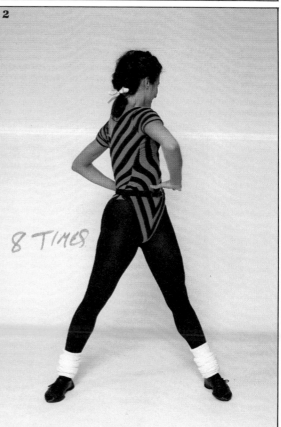

8 TIMES

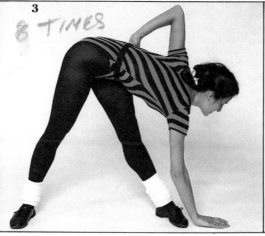

8 TIMES

Twist and toe touches

1 *Stand with your feet a little over hip distance apart, hands on your waist.*
2 *Twist to the left from the waist only, not from the hips, keeping feet flat on ground.*
3 *Bend over from the waist and extend your right arm to the floor or to touch your left foot, keeping your left elbow bent. Come up centre and reverse, twisting and bending to the right. Repeat 8 times. Aim to get your hand flat on the floor eventually.*

Abdominals

These exercises are designed specially to strengthen your upper, middle and lower abdominal muscles and to burn up any excess fat in this area. Don't try and cheat on these exercises or you will not receive any benefits from them.

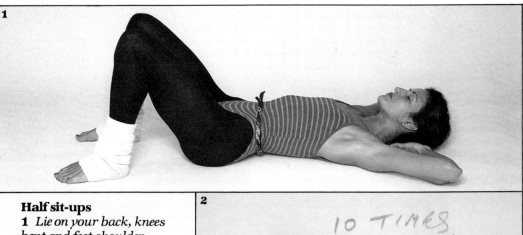

Half sit-ups

1 *Lie on your back, knees bent and feet shoulder distance apart. Clasp your hands behind your head.*
2 *Raise your upper body and head off the floor, pulling up with stomach muscles only. Hold for a count of 4, lower slowly. Hold for 4 counts, not touching floor. Repeat 10 times.*

10 TIMES.

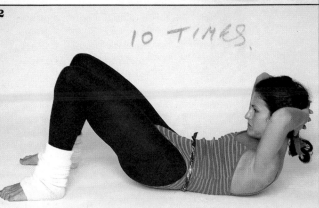

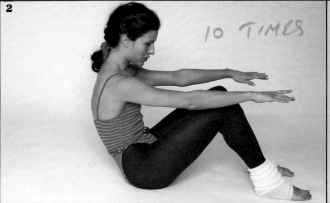

10 TIMES

Full sit-ups

1 *Lie on your back with your knees bent and feet shoulder distance apart. Raise your head and upper body off the floor and then extend your arms.*
2 *Roll up into a sitting position, exhaling as you do so. Roll down again without head and shoulders touching the floor and inhale. Repeat 10 times.*

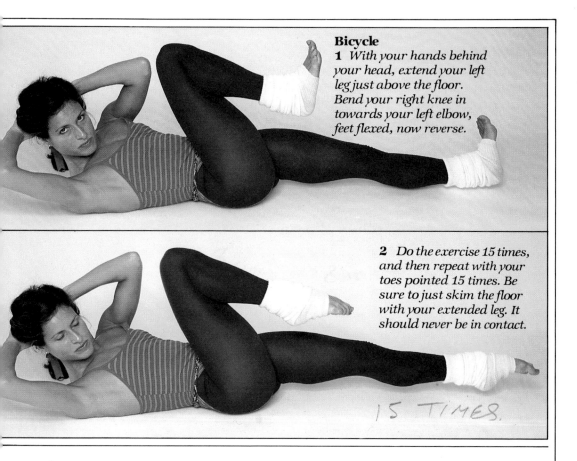

Bicycle
1 *With your hands behind your head, extend your left leg just above the floor. Bend your right knee in towards your left elbow, feet flexed, now reverse.*

2 *Do the exercise 15 times, and then repeat with your toes pointed 15 times. Be sure to just skim the floor with your extended leg. It should never be in contact.*

15 TIMES.

Backs

This exercise is good for releasing the abdominal muscles at the end of this section of the work-out as well as strengthening your back muscles and removing tension from the lower back area. It is therapeutic if you have back pain.

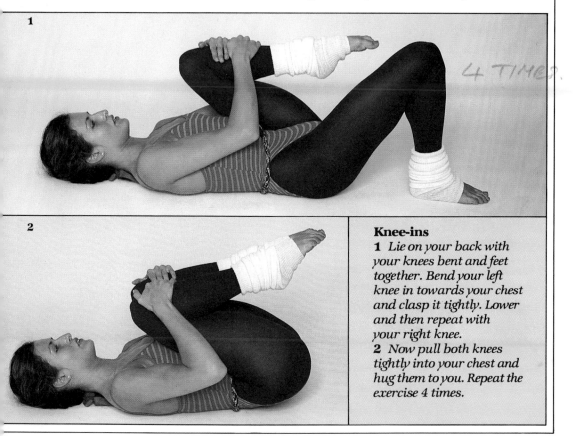

1

4 TIMES.

2

Knee-ins
1 *Lie on your back with your knees bent and feet together. Bend your left knee in towards your chest and clasp it tightly. Lower and then repeat with your right knee.*
2 *Now pull both knees tightly into your chest and hug them to you. Repeat the exercise 4 times.*

Hips and thighs

These exercises aim at trimming and toning your hip and thigh muscles and are particularly effective for strengthening the inner thighs which are often slack and inclined to run to fat on many women. Performed in sequence regularly, they will help tone up your front, outer, back and inner thigh muscles.

Front leg kick

Lie on your back, legs together and arms at your sides. Raise your right leg as high as it will go 8 times. Now reverse and raise the left leg 8 times, keeping your toes pointed and back flat on the floor.

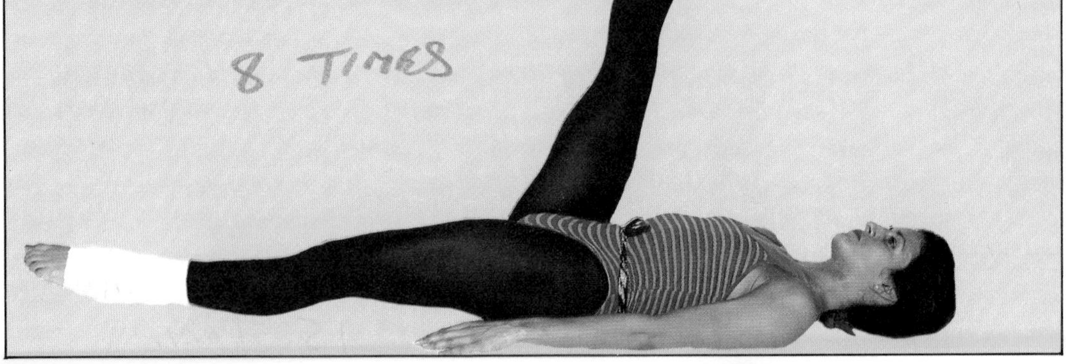

8 TIMES

1

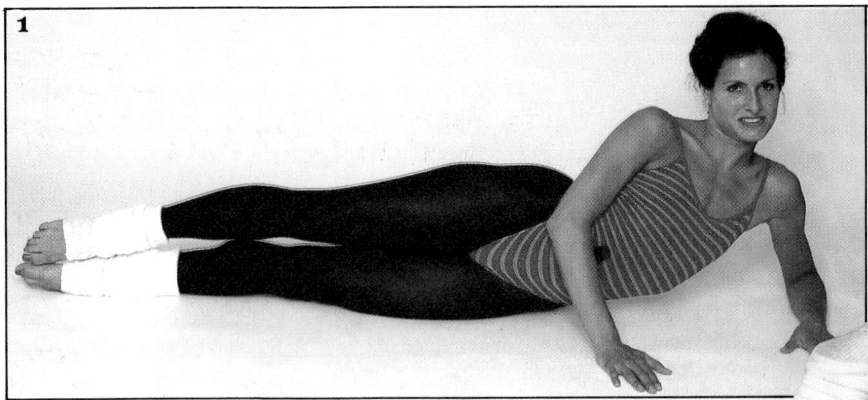

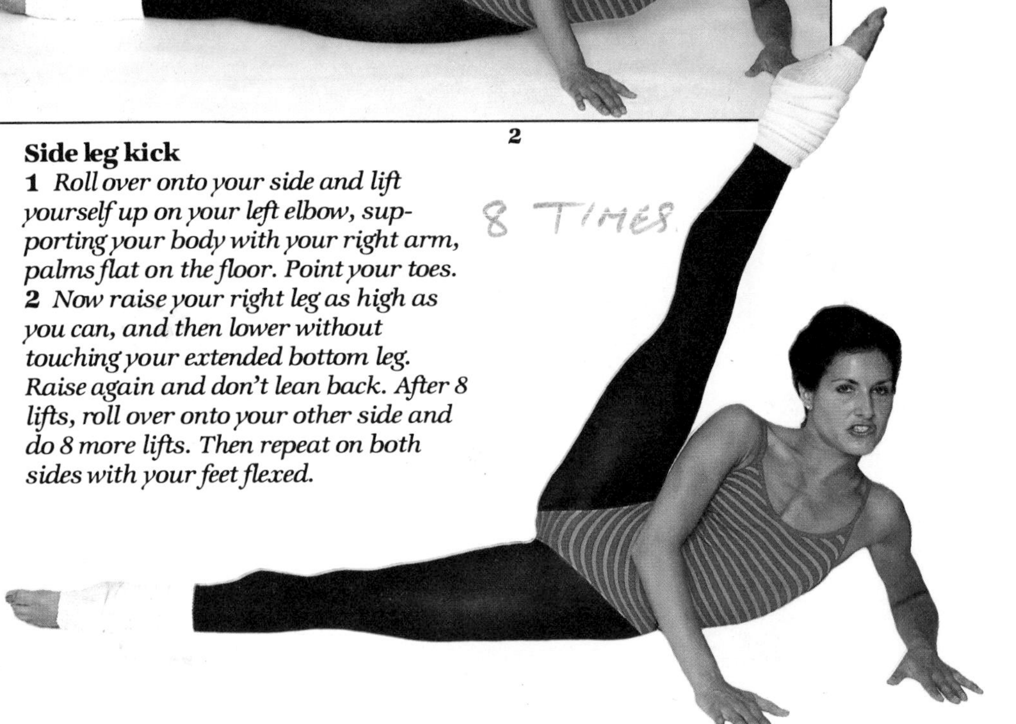

Side leg kick

2

1 *Roll over onto your side and lift yourself up on your left elbow, supporting your body with your right arm, palms flat on the floor. Point your toes.*
2 *Now raise your right leg as high as you can, and then lower without touching your extended bottom leg. Raise again and don't lean back. After 8 lifts, roll over onto your other side and do 8 more lifts. Then repeat on both sides with your feet flexed.*

8 TIMES

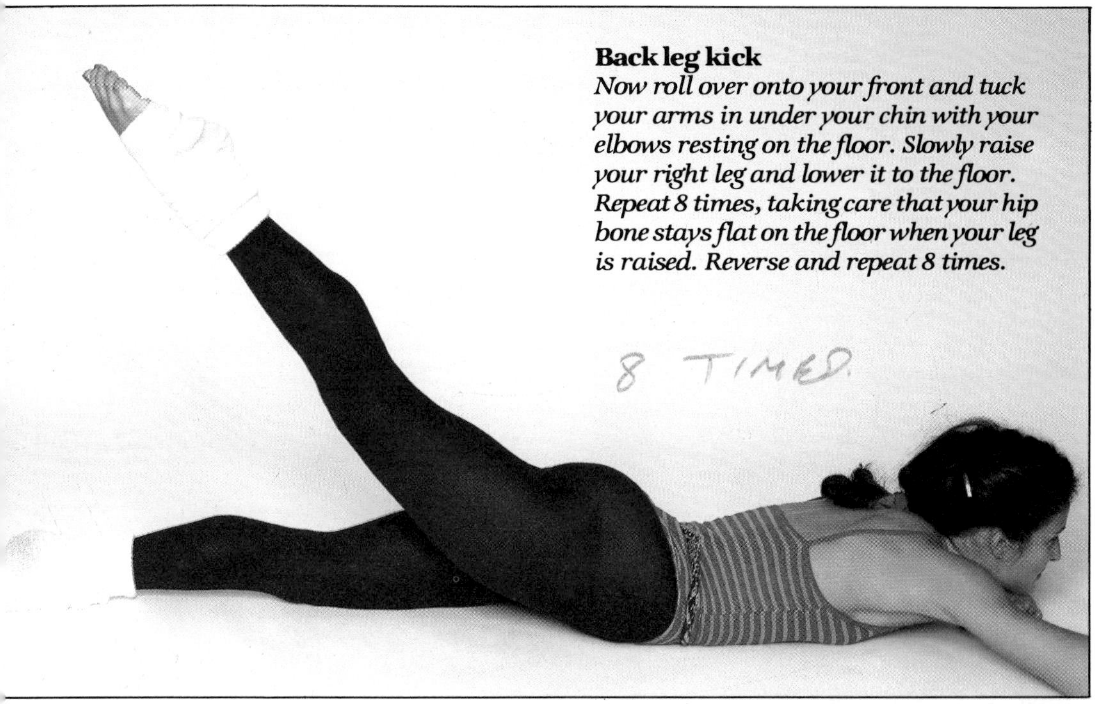

Back leg kick

Now roll over onto your front and tuck your arms in under your chin with your elbows resting on the floor. Slowly raise your right leg and lower it to the floor. Repeat 8 times, taking care that your hip bone stays flat on the floor when your leg is raised. Reverse and repeat 8 times.

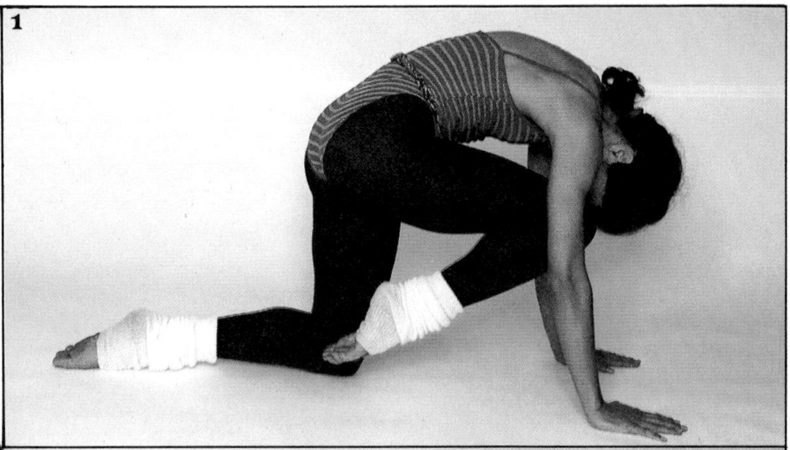

8 TIMES.

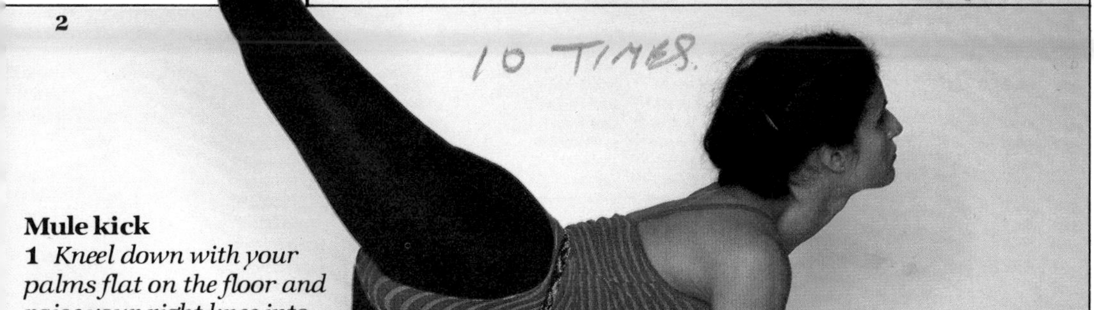

10 TIMES.

Mule kick

1 Kneel down with your palms flat on the floor and raise your right knee into chin with head tucked in.
2 Stretch leg out backwards as far as it will go and stretch out your neck. Repeat 10 times each leg.

Hips and thighs *continued*

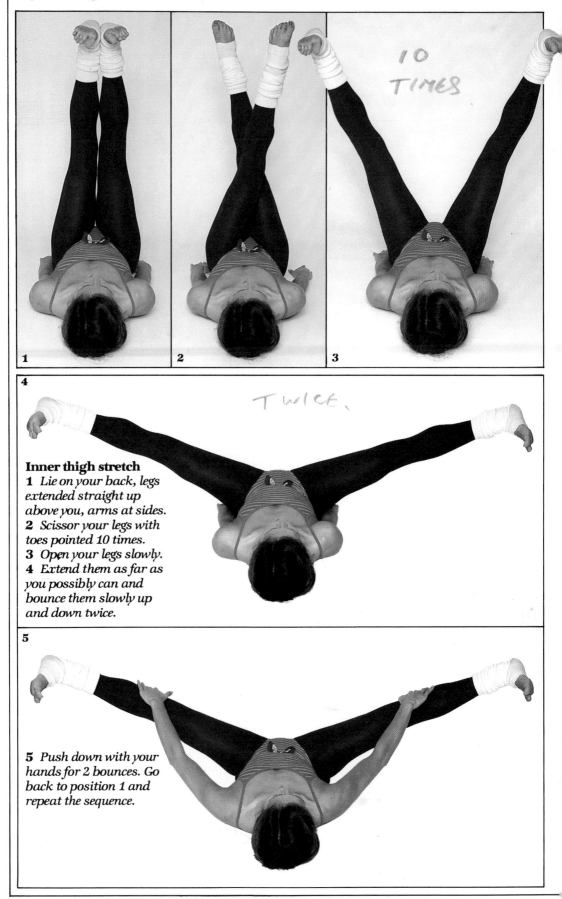

10 TIMES

1

2

3

4

TWICE.

Inner thigh stretch
1 *Lie on your back, legs extended straight up above you, arms at sides.*
2 *Scissor your legs with toes pointed 10 times.*
3 *Open your legs slowly.*
4 *Extend them as far as you possibly can and bounce them slowly up and down twice.*

5

5 *Push down with your hands for 2 bounces. Go back to position 1 and repeat the sequence.*

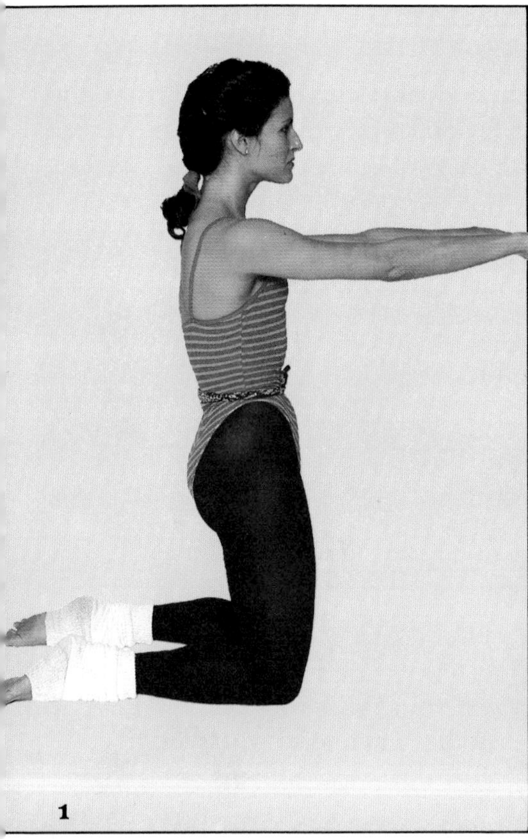

Quadriceps stretch
1 *Kneel on the floor with back straight and arms extended, stomach in.*
2 *Slowly lean back, with back straight, as far as you can go for 4 counts. Come back up for 4 counts. Repeat 10 times.*

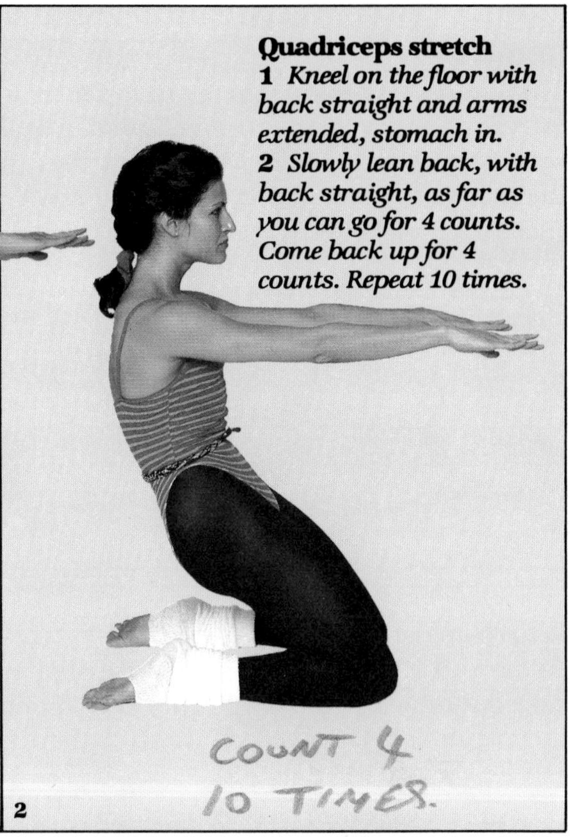

1

2

COUNT 4
10 TIMES.

1

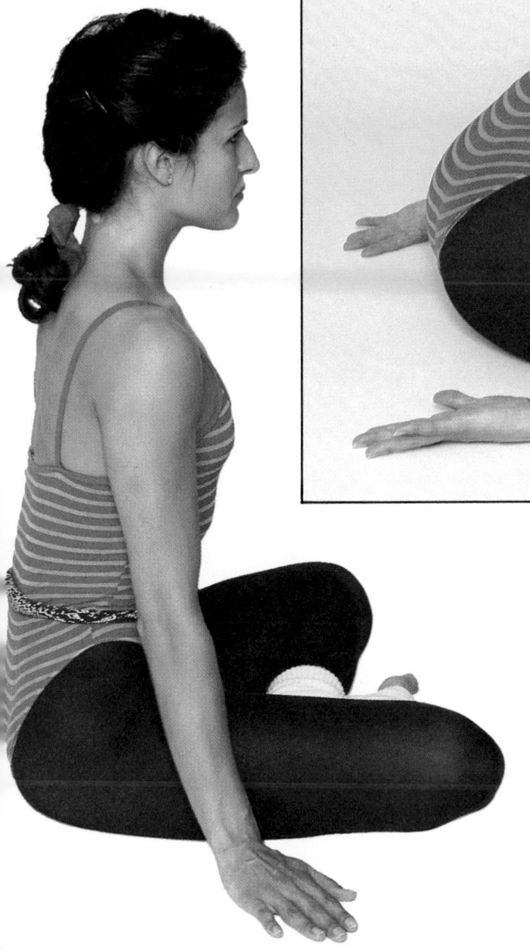

2

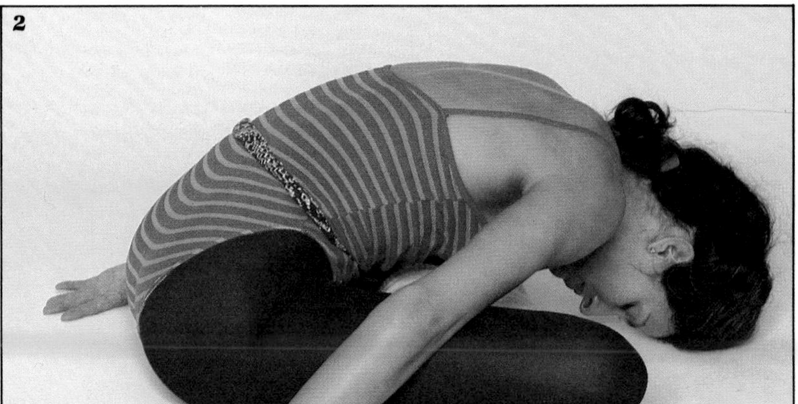

Hip and thigh release
1 *Sit cross-legged on the floor with your back straight and arms at your sides, your palms flat on the floor.*
2 *Now roll down over your legs extending your arms back behind you. Hold for a count of 10 and then roll up slowly.*

1 TIME
COUNT 10

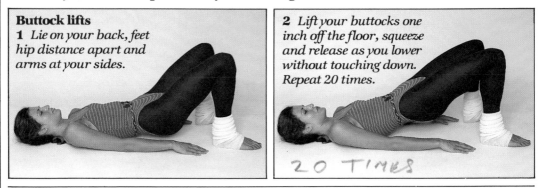

Buttocks

This exercise will tone up the muscles in your buttocks, making them firmer and burning up any fatty deposits. You can make it harder as you get more advanced by bringing your knees together in the centre as you squeeze and then opening them as you relax. Repeat with your feet together. Here is the basic exercise.

Buttock lifts
1 *Lie on your back, feet hip distance apart and arms at your sides.*

2 *Lift your buttocks one inch off the floor, squeeze and release as you lower without touching down. Repeat 20 times.*

Warm-down

At the end of your work-out it is essential to do a few gentle stretching exercises to ease out muscles and help your body to relax and your pulse rate to slow down to its normal level. Don't rush through them — do them in a leisurely way.

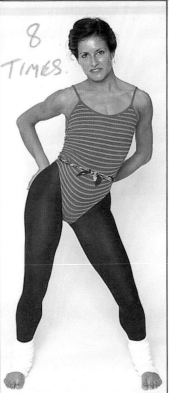

Hip circles
Stand with your feet shoulder distance apart, hands resting on your hips. With knees slightly bent, swing from side to side, backwards and forwards and then in circles for 8 counts each.

Ceiling kiss
1 *Stand with hands on your waist and your feet hip distance apart, head bent slightly forwards over your body.*
2 *Stretch both your head and neck backwards as far as you can for a count of 8 and then lower again for 8 counts. This will tighten up your neck muscles.*

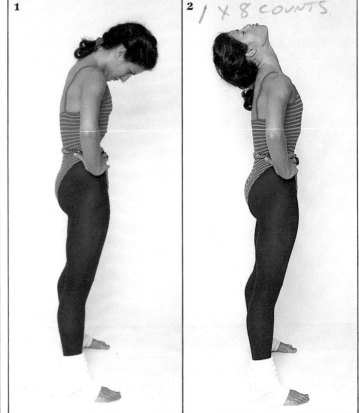

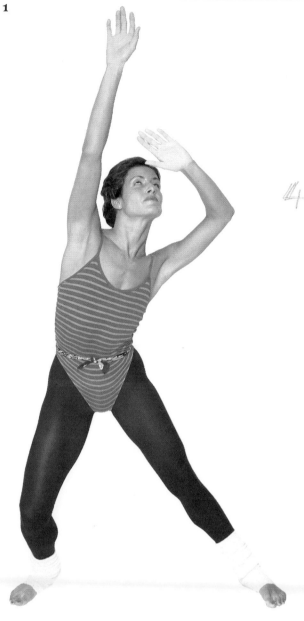

1

4

Special body stretch
1 *Stand with your feet a little over hip distance apart and lunge to the right with your right knee bent and left leg extended, raising your right arm and bending your left. Reverse and repeat 4 times, stretching up really high.*
2 *Now lean over and bounce down slowly with your arms crossed as low as you can go for 4 counts.*
3 *Swing your arms out to the left, and repeat 4 times, dragging your hands along the floor. Return to the centre and roll up very slowly, one vertebra at a time, until you are upright. Congratulations! You have completed your first work-out.*

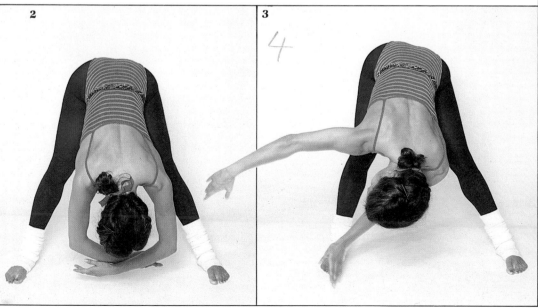

2

3

4

Working-out with weights

Weight-training is becoming more popular with women who want to stay fit and slim, for far from building up ugly muscle bulk, it can make you firmer and leaner. If practised properly with light weights you can decrease heavy areas of your body and maintain or increase areas which need more mass. Because you have high levels of oestrogen and little of the male hormone testosterone in your body, you cannot develop large bulky muscles. You can either train in a gym with proper dumb-bells or work-out at home with cans of soup, books or telephone directories — they are all suitable. Most women start out with 1.25kg weights and progress to 2.50kg or more as they become fitter and stronger. You can purchase weights for use at home in many good sports shops. Weight-training brings many benefits, including increased fitness and strength for other forms of exercise and sport, and well-conditioned muscles which burn more calories at rest to keep you slim. Like any other form of exercise, always warm-up for five or 10 minutes before you start working-out to prepare your heart and lungs and to increase blood supply to your muscles. Follow the exercises in the work-out warm-up and aerobic sections (see pages 94-97). Wear something loose and comfortable such as shorts and a T-shirt or a tracksuit to allow maximum unrestricted movement.

1

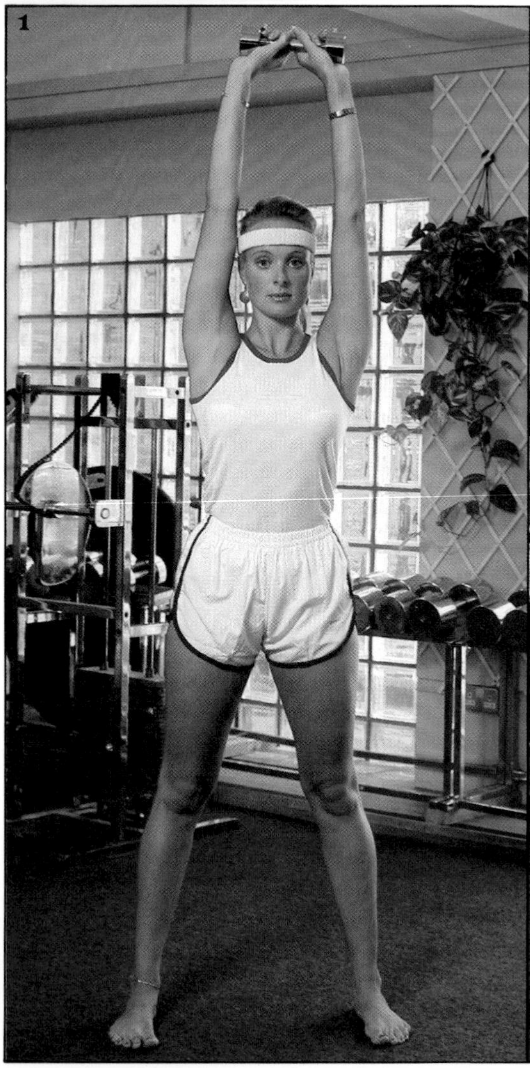

Warm-up swings
1 *This exercise will warm-up muscles. Stand with feet shoulder distance apart, arms outstretched above your head, holding weights in both hands.*
2 *Bending knees, with arms straight, swing them down between your legs. Raise again and repeat 10 times.*

2

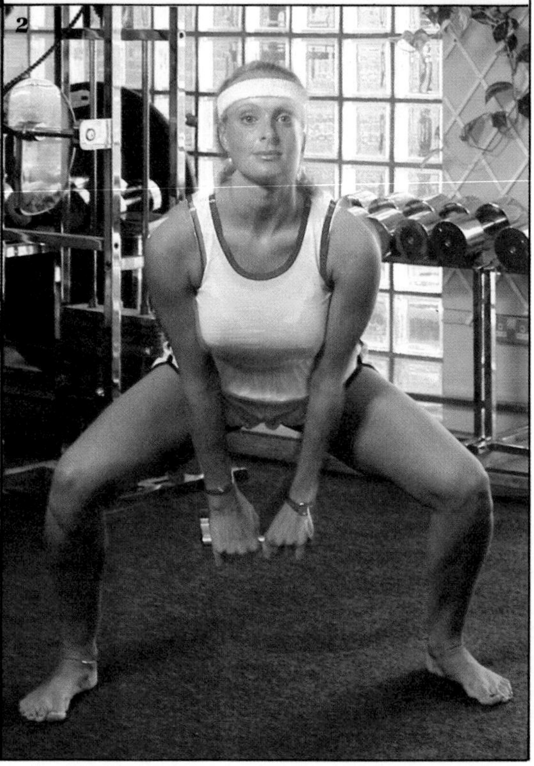

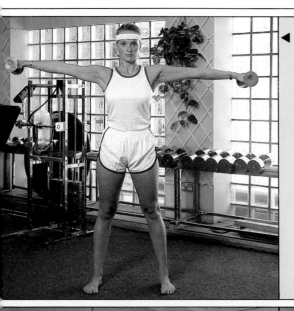

◄ **Side lifts**
Stand with feet shoulder-distance apart, arms outstretched straight at shoulder height, holding a weight in each hand. Slowly lower arms to your sides and raise again. Repeat 10 times. This is good for strengthening upper arms.

French curls
1 Stand with feet shoulder distance apart, arms above head, holding weight downwards between your palms.
2 Bend your elbows and lower weight behind your head. Slowly raise arms again above head. Repeat 10 times. This is good for firming backs of arms.
▼

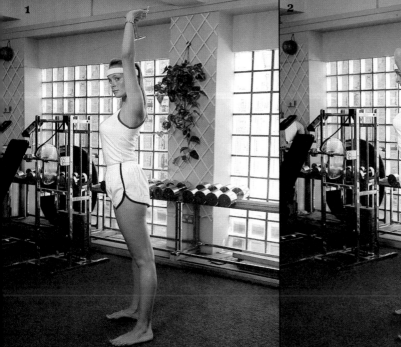

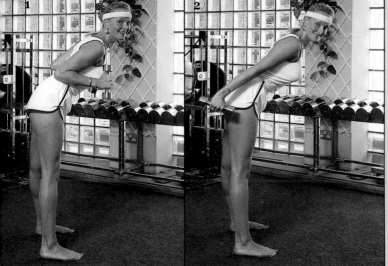

Triceps extension
1 With feet shoulder distance apart, lean slightly forwards with back straight. Hold a weight in each hand with arms bent close to sides.
2 Keeping your back straight at the same angle, extend your arms backwards from the elbows. They should be parallel to the sides of your body. Slowly raise your lower arms and repeat 10 times. Good for flabby under-arms.

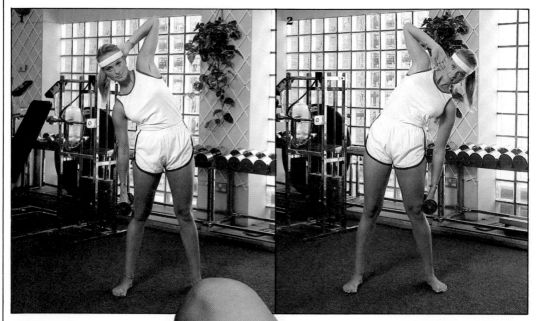

Side bends

1 *Stand with feet shoulder distance apart, left arm bent with hand behind head. Hold the weight in your right hand. Lean over from the waist to the right so that right arm is lowered. Come up slowly repeat 10 times.*
2 *Reverse and, holding weight in left hand, lean over to the left. Come up slowly and repeat 10 times.*

Supine bench press

1 *See opposite above. Lie on bench with knees bent, feet flat on bench. Bend your arms on each side, holding a weight in each hand.*
2 *Breathe out and raise arms up above head and extend them straight up. Breathe in and lower. Repeat 10 times. Good for chest.*

All the exercises shown are for firming the upper body only from the waist upwards, although you can buy special strap-on leg weights for toning up leg muscles too. When you work-out with weights you are adding stress to an exercise to make your body work even harder. Consequently, your muscles will eventually become stronger and with increased endurance, and your body will look leaner with more pronounced contours. Weight-training is an excellent way of eliminating cellulite on under-arms too. Remember to breathe deeply as you perform the exercises, inhaling as you lower the weights and exhaling as you raise them, as a general rule.

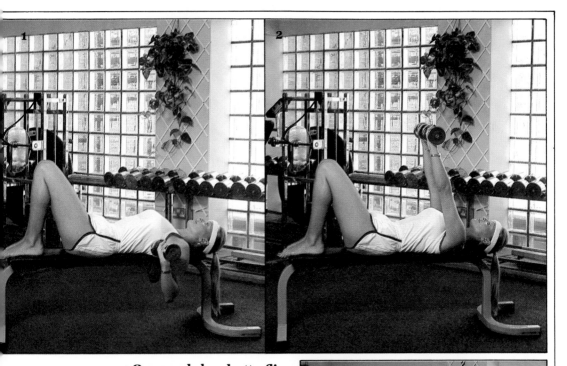

Open and close butterflies

1 *Lie on bench with knees bent and feet flat. Raise your arms above chest with elbows bent and hands touching in centre, a weight in each.*
2 *Slowly open your arms to the sides, keeping your elbows slightly bent. Hold for a count of 3 and then slowly bring arms into centre again. Repeat 10 times. Good for firming pectoral muscles.*

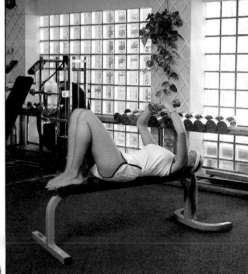

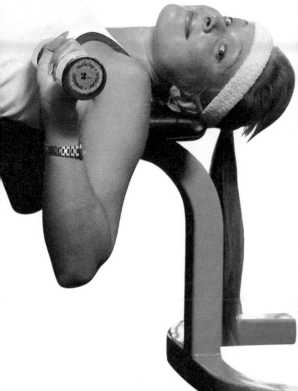

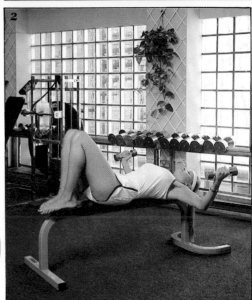

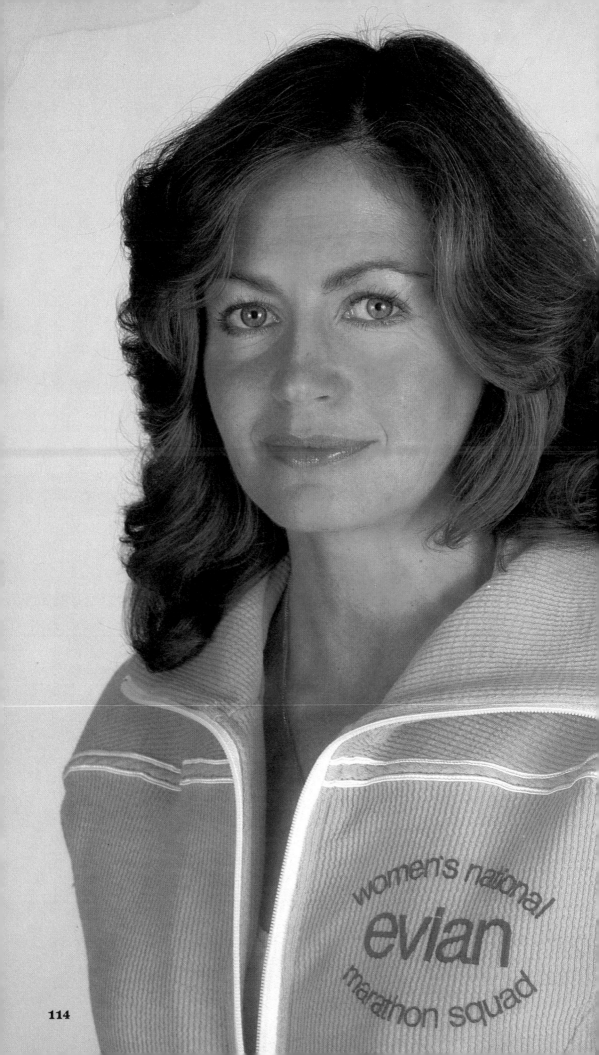

HEALTH & BEAUTY PROFILE

Leslie Watson

When you first meet slim, dark haired Leslie Watson you might be forgiven for mistaking her for a glamorous model but really she is one of Britain's top marathon runners and the women's 50 mile world record holder. A busy state registerd physiotherapist with her own practice in London's West End, Leslie runs between 60 and 100 miles per week in training and is a firm believer in looking good as well as feeling good.

Before a big race she always makes up carefully, washes her hair, does her nails and puts tanning lotion on her legs to make them look even slimmer. She feels that this give her the confidence to do well. She always uses a good conditioner on her hair and has it permed and highlighted regularly at a top London salon. Her skincare routine is very simple: "I have naturally dry skin and need to use moisturising cream. I use pure unscented soap and water."

Leslie started running in her home town of Glasgow when she was 10. She thought that she had no natural talent for athletics and only joined a local club when a friend told her that there was a girl who trained there who was almost as slow as her! However, under the guidance of top coach John Anderson she went on to make the Scottish team and to win the women's Scottish cross-country and one-mile track events in the mid-1960s. She has been running marathons regularly since 1975.

She is living proof that women can succeed in sport without losing their femininity and thinks that because of their hormanal make-up: "It is terribly difficult for women to put on muscle." Her advice to women who start running is: "Take it easy at the start and don't be put off initially by thinking 'I can't do it'. You can if you just keep on trying. Even people who have no natural talent can go in for endurance sports if they are dedicated and train regularly." As a physiotherapist she believes that many running injuries are caused by wearing the wrong footwear and thinks that good running shoes are always a worthwhile investment.

Leslie thinks that natural wholefoods are best and advises all women to eat them. "I would never buy anything other than 100 per cent wholemeal bread, and I hardly ever eat meat, only fish. I like vegetarian food best of all but there are so few good vegetarian restaurants and I eat out a lot. I always eat a good breakfast because mentally it puts me in a good mood. I take multi-vitamin tablets every day plus one gram of vitamin E, two to three grams of vitamin C, vitamin B1 and evening primrose oil." However, despite her healthy eating habits she admits that sweet things are a great temptation to her. "I just can't resist them, and I eat too much chocolate. I have no will-power when it comes to eating and that's why I have to run! If I ate less, I'm sure I would run better." But burning up calories at the rate she does when she's out running, it's no wonder Leslie manages to look so slim.

As well as running, Leslie has a busy working schedule, is presently involved in making a film on running marathons and holds regular physiotherapy clinics for fellow runners at a chain of London running shops. She relaxes by going out running but says "I also like to read, go to the theatre and aerobic classes.'

To Leslie, running has become a way of life and keeps her fit and healthy. "I think that running and vitamins help prevent me getting ill and that's why I never have anything wrong with me."

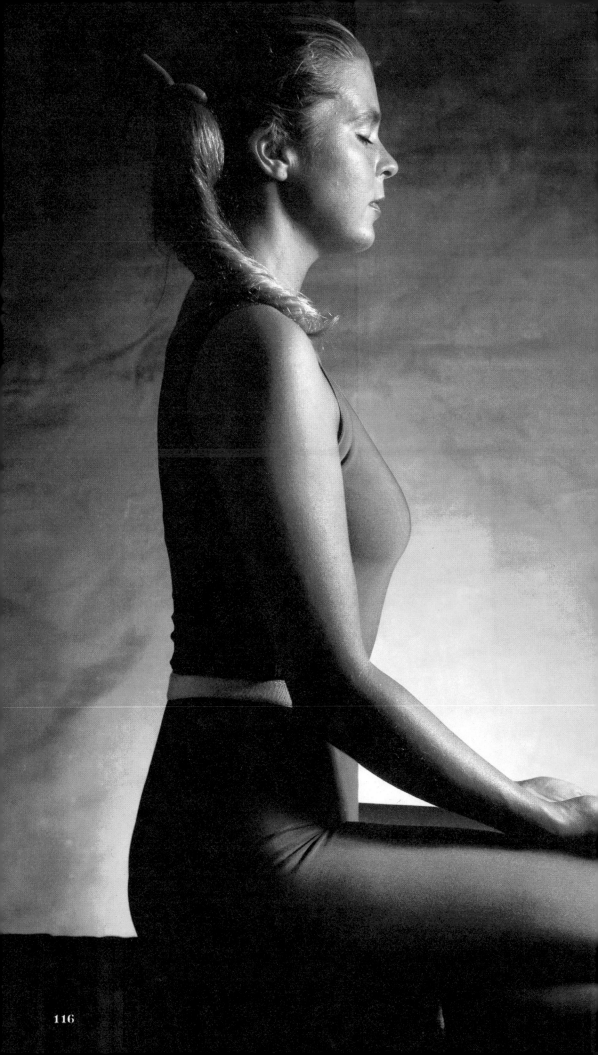

TAKING IT EASY

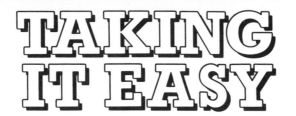

If you want to be really fit and healthy, you must look after your mind as well as your body, for relaxation and exercise are equally important for integrated beauty, health and fitness. Whereas physical activity can help alleviate body stress and promote a strong heart and muscles and supple limbs, relaxation and mental activity can reduce emotional stress and help you to think more clearly and objectively. They are different sides of the same coin and it is vital that you realise this and make time for relaxing in your campaign to get fit. After all, your body and mind are fused — they do not exist independently of each other — and it is important to reach a mental peak in addition to your maximum physical potential.

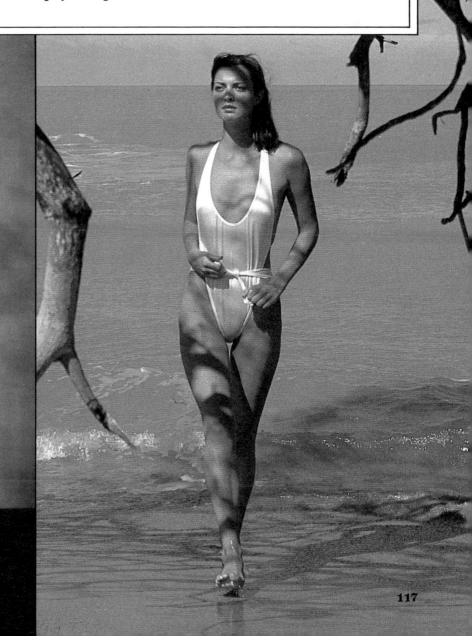

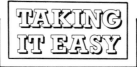

We live in a fast-moving, highly technological world and often we become
alienated from our true selves and subject
to stress. Psychologists reckon that most of
us are too tense and that many
psychosomatic illnesses are triggered off
by our inability to cope with the pressures
of modern-day living. Our bodies were
not specifically designed to handle these
and the reaction of many overworked
doctors is to prescribe tranquillisers and
other drugs when their patients complain
of worries at work and at home. However,
drugs can only treat the symptoms of
nervous tension — they cannot remove
the causes. We can take positive steps to
teach ourselves how to consciously
monitor our reactions to stress and how to
cut off safely before it takes its toll on our
minds and bodies.

The best and most effective way of
relaxing is to learn a special technique,
such as deep breathing, meditation or
yoga. Flopping down in a chair in front of
the television after a busy, tiring day is not
necessarily relaxing, for to relax mentally
you must relax your body too and it may
be stiff and tense with aching muscles.
Flaking out or simply falling asleep
through sheer tiredness will not yield
positive results nor will you necessarily
feel fresh and revitalised afterwards.
However, you can train yourself to relax
in such a way that your heartbeat is
lowered, your oxygen consumption
decreased as you breathe more slowly
and regularly, and even your brainwave
patterns are changed. Afterwards, you will
feel more energetic and fulfilled.

When you relax consciously and deeply
you become more aware of your body
and your own inner life. You may find
that it is a creative time when you can
experience new ideas and can make
important decisions concerning your
work, family and friendships. This is a
way of getting to know yourself better and
discovering a new sense of stillness and
serenity as you feel the tension gradually
flowing out of your body. It may not come
naturally to you at first and it will take
practice, especially if you are one of those
hyperactive people who always has to be
doing something and finds it difficult to
slow down, even for a few minutes. But

relaxation is not a waste of time; rather, it
is a positive way of making more time for
yourself by providing more energy for
other tasks and activities. Do not feel guilty
that you are 'not doing anything' when
you set aside a fixed time each day for
relaxation. On the contrary, you are
recharging your body's batteries and
guarding against stress. You will soon
come to enjoy these quiet moments in a
day and to look forward to them as a time
for reflection and contemplation. Make it
an unbreakable habit and do the same
exercises every day at a convenient time.
You may prefer the mornings before you
get up and leave for work, or perhaps in
the evenings after a stressful day or last
thing at night before you go to bed. The
time is not important provided that you
make it a regular date.

Perhaps the most important function of
relaxation is that it can teach you to take
control of your life and enables you to
channel it into the direction you wish to
go. You no longer feel the victim of
circumstances or a pawn in the hands of
greater forces as you develop more power
over your own life and improve your
creative potential. You will feel more
confident about your abilities and more
contented within yourself. Many people
also experience greater powers of
concentration as you learn to focus their
minds more clearly. They may find also
that their memory improves after years of
forgetfulness and confused thinking.
Therefore at work or at home you can
function at the height of your intellectual
and emotional powers.

Many people find that regular physical
exercise, especially of the aerobic kind
such as endurance running or cycling, is
an effective way of relaxing. Even after a
demanding run they feel refreshed and
exhilarated with new energy. While they
exercise they become conscious of the
inner workings of their bodies and block
out their external stimuli and surround-
ings, preferring to think creative thoughts
and to sort out any problems or worries
that they might have. Some even experience what has become known as the
'runners's high' — a sense of floating and
euphoria as they seem to enter a higher
plane. There is no doubt that rhythmic

exercise can be pleasantly tranquillising and therapeutic, enabling you to escape from the pressures of everyday life and enjoy a wonderful sense of freedom and release from tension. You might be tired before you exercise but you will feel totally restored and relaxed afterwards. You will feel less tense and stressful, any problems you may have will become less significant and your body will also seem more relaxed and supple. But it is still a good idea to supplement your exercise with a relaxation technique. Yoga is particularly effective as it helps relax muscle groups and other areas of the body that may be tightened by some forms of strenuous exercise.

Stress

Your body is rather like a clock — if you overwind it, it will start to run down and may even stop eventually. We tend to overwind ourselves every day — rushing to meet deadlines or to finish the job, coping with domestic problems, managing a busy demanding schedule all contribute to stress. Sometimes it is necessary to unwind and turn off, whether it's a holiday away from it all, a run in the park, a swim in the pool, a regular yoga session or 15 minutes' meditation. The level of stress to which we are exposed is highly individual, of course, and depends to a great extent on our lifestyle, our emotional relationships, the nature of our work and our temperament. Stress is a contributory factor in many 'affluent' illnesses, especially heart disease, ulcers, depression and mental illness. Our bodies and minds react to stressful situations by becoming tense, and unless we can channel this tension into safe outlets, such as relaxation and meditation, it may trigger off serious physical and nervous disorders, ranging from insomnia, asthma and migraine to high blood pressure, heart disease and strokes.

There are different kinds of stress which you may encounter in your life — emotional, physiological and environmental. Emotional stress is probably the most common and it may stem from something as trivial as a quarrel or as serious as a marriage breakdown and divorce, or even the death of a friend or member of the family. Divorce is one of the most stressful experiences that people can undergo in their lives and American studies have shown that newly divorced people are 10 times more likely to become ill than are married or traditionally single people. As the divorce rate rises and a third of marriages break up, emotional stress is bound to become more common. Physiological stress is triggered off by the release of steroid hormones from the adrenal glands, whereas environmental stress, caused by excessive heat or cold, is physical and requires medical treatment.

Most stress is caused by changes in our lives — especially our work, our personal relationships or our living arrangements. We each have our own level of tolerance and when we pass beyond this we may become physically or emotionally ill. Our emotional state can affect our muscles, making them tense so that in time they shorten. Later when we try to stretch them they may get damaged or tear. And the more physically inactive you are, the higher your neuromuscular tension, your pulse rate and your blood pressure making you a prime candidate for modern stress-related diseases.

When your body is subjected to stress, it undergoes physiological changes — your bloodstream is flooded with adrenalin, your blood pressure rises, your muscles flex, you may start to sweat and your whole body will feel tense. Fear, guilt, overwork, worry can all cause your heart to start racing and the onset of these unpleasant symptoms. Even when they subside, you are often left with an aching head or back, and feeling tired or even giddy. Often there is no way of avoiding these situations, but you can learn to make stress work positively in your favour by responding confidently and decisively instead of reacting negatively. Anger and tears are the usual release valves and although many people appear to respond calmly enough on the surface, in reality they bottle up their emotions inside and become unhappy and tense. However, you can train yourself to release nervous tension and to harness the energy forces of stress to your advantage, thus reducing its psychological and physical effects.

But first, to come to terms with stress, you must understand a little about your nervous system and how your body responds. The two branches of the nervous system, the parasympathetic and sympathetic systems, are made up of nerve fibres which radiate out from the spine throughout your body. Whereas the

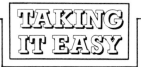
parasympathetic branch relaxes your muscles, lowers your heartbeat and generally relaxes your body, helping you to breathe more slowly and restfully as air flow to your lungs is reduced, the sympathetic branch usually takes over when you are under stress, causing adrenalin to be pumped into the blood, your heart to beat faster, your arteries to contract and blood pressure to rise. In other words, it prepares your body for action, rather like an animal when it is challenged or threatened. Your body becomes tense as the blood containing fat and sugar energy from metabolism is rushed to your muscles and then, like an animal, you are ready to fight or run away from your aggressor or challenge. This is a perfectly normal reaction and is nothing to worry about in itself. However, if it happens frequently over a long period it can be damaging to your health and make you more vulnerable to disease as your immune response to stress ceases to function. Your muscles and major organs (heart, lungs, kidneys and liver) become tense and your circulatory system is affected. Your body starts to age more rapidly and is more likely to fall prey to degenerative diseases, high blood pressure, arthritis and even cancer.

The stressful condition should not last long however and your body should soon return to normal as heart rate decreases to its resting rate and your breathing slows down. You soon stop sweating, and normal functioning is resumed. However, your muscles may still feel tense, your nerves on edge, your head may ache and you will not feel relaxed. When the parasympathetic branch is dominant your mind and body will be in harmony and you will feel rested and serene. Of course, you cannot spend your life avoiding stress. On the contrary, many ambitious people who love their work seem to thrive on stress, both intellectually and emotionally. To them, stress is enjoyable and challenging, and provided that they have the capacity to relax and unwind afterwards they can make it a rewarding part of their lives which helps them to fulfill their individual potential. It makes their lives more interesting and enriches them in their work and their relations with other people. They enjoy the thrill of the adrenalin and feel more energetic as a result. If you number yourself among these people and have a sedentary office job, you must be sure to find a physical outlet for this increased energy — sports and exercise are perfect and relaxing. Ideally, both branches of your nervous system should be balanced so that you can enjoy the pressures of work and respond positively to stress but still have the ability to relax afterwards and feel restored without suffering from long-term tension.

We all have these resources to cope with stress even if we do not all possess the same stress threshold. Nobody can live under constant stress without suffering from high blood pressure or hypertension eventually, so learn to handle each new challenge as it comes along and how to switch off and relieve tension so that you do not become generally fatigued. Firstly, try treating stress situations as a challenge and enjoy them calmly, removing the ones that are not useful or fulfilling. Start by looking at your work. Is it satisfying? Do you enjoy it? Are there areas that you could change for the better? Then examine other stressful areas in your life and try to cancel out any negative ones. Establish a positive relationship with stress and use

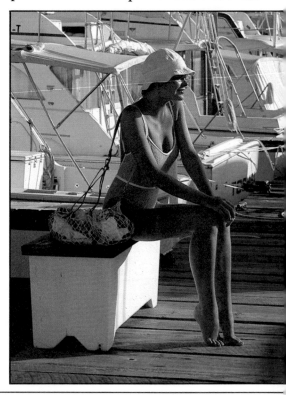

it; don't fight it or run away from it. Be strong and make it an exciting and interesting part of your life.

And as a contrast, make time for relaxation, by practising yoga or meditation or a special breathing technique or by exercise — running, cycling, swimming, playing tennis, joining a gym or a work-out class. They will all help channel your energy and add an extra dimension to your life, which you will come to enjoy. Hobbies and leisure interests can help you to unwind, and they too play their part in relieving tension. If you are feeling tense, try going for a walk or jog, doing some gardening or painting, playing the piano or enjoying your favourite sport. They will help take your mind off any problems you may have and enable you to think more clearly about them.

In 1976, the New York Academy of Sciences stated that endurance runners who run long distances in training each week tend to be less anxious and more emotionally stable than their physically

Most people relax and escape from stress by getting away from it all on holiday. A break from work and your usual routine will help you unwind, and anxieties and worries will assume less troubling proportions as you relax on the beach or quayside, or just float in the swimming pool.

inactive contemporaries. In fact, many doctors are coming to realise that regular physical exercise can encourage self-confidence and release negative stressful emotions and tension. Many people discover a new sense of purpose in exercise with new goals to aim at and achieve. Their sense of being ultimately in control of their own lives tends to diminish the negative impact of stress on their bodies and exercise becomes necessary for their emotional as well as their physical health.

Diet and stress

Your diet can also help combat stress and make you more alert and energetic in your everyday life. A poor diet that is high in fats and sugars and lacks essential vitamins and minerals can contribute to general fatigue, tension and even depression. The B-complex vitamins are necessary for maintaining a healthy nervous system. For example, the vitamin B_{12} (cyanocobalamin) helps protect you against insomnia, depression and fatigue. Found in organ meats, wheat germ, meat, egg yolks and some fish, it helps in the metabolism of fats, protein and carbohydrates. Without it you will feel tired and listless and your memory will most probably become poor. This is the vitamin that many vegetarians tend to be deficient in, and it is important that they take it as a supplement to their diet. Other B vitamins

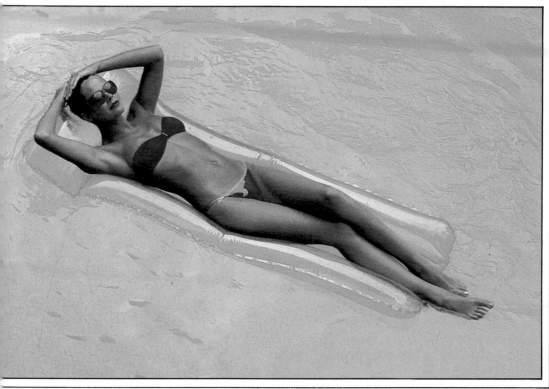

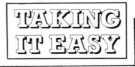

for promoting mental health include B2 (riboflavin) which protects your adrenal glands, and also pantothenic acid which fights stress and increases your resistance to it. Both of these vitamins are found in organ meats, brewers yeast and legumes. If you are eating a healthy wholefoods diet that contains plenty of fresh fruit and vegetables, meat and fish, whole grain cereals and legumes you should be getting an adequate supply of all these essential nutrients.

Relaxation techniques

There are special techniques that you can learn to use to induce a relaxed mental and physical state. By consciously training yourself to relax in this way you can eliminate tension from your mind and body. And just lying down is not relaxing in itself if your mind is in turmoil, as this tension will be transmitted throughout your body and you will feel stiff and tense. The way you breathe can also help to clear your consciousness and make you feel calm and restful. In both meditation and yoga, breathing is the key to changing your mood and energy level. Thus when you are tense, angry or anxious you tend to breathe quickly in small shallow gasps. Breathing in this way does not allow sufficient oxygen to be absorbed into the bloodstream, and thus the amount available for meeting the needs of your heart and other organs, brain, nerves and skin is restricted and your body fails to function efficiently. Because your nerve cells and brain are short of oxygen you may start to feel tired and low in spirits.

However, the opposite is true when you relax — you tend to breathe more slowly and deeply, inhaling more oxygen to supply your body's needs and to expel waste matter from your system. You feel more comfortable, calmer, your vitality is increased and you have more energy thanks to higher levels of oxygen in your bloodstream, cells and tissues. Try it when you next feel angry, nervous or upset — deliberately breathe more slowly, taking in deep lungfuls of air and breathing with your whole chest and abdomen. You will soon begin to feel calmer as the oxygen gets to work.

We cannot live without oxygen as it is necessary for the correct functioning of nearly all our body processes. It fuels our bodies and gives us energy, just like the food we eat. The air we breathe contains oxygen, nitrogen, inert gases (argon, krypton, xenon, helium and neon), water moisture and traces of mineral salts. When we inhale, we take air down into our lungs from whence oxygen is absorbed into the bloodstream for use by the body. When we exhale, we expel carbon dioxide, the by-product of oxidation, and wastes. However, if we do not exhale fully, some of these waste materials are retained in the system and they may eventually contribute to disease and ageing. There is no doubt that some chest disorders can improve if full breathing is taught.

Most religions and philosophies at different times throughout the world's history have accorded breathing a very special significance. It is traditionally associated with power and energy. Thus in the Bible the Holy Spirit is the breath of God. In fact, the Latin word for breath is *spiritus*, and the definition of 'spirit' is the life force that animates the bodies of living things. Thus there can be no life without breath. The Chinese call it *chi*, whereas the yogis refer to it as *prana* and harness it in their meditation to control their minds and even to overcome pain itself. By developing your lung capacity to the full you too can improve your health and feel more energetic and revitalised. Use one of the following breathing techniques, yoga or meditation to supplement your aerobic exercise which can give you even greater heart-lung capacity and also cardiovascular fitness.

Breathing

Start by lying flat on your back on the floor or a hard level surface. A carpet, rug or towel will help make you feel more comfortable. Always wear some loose unrestricting clothing so that your body is not tightly enclosed or inhibited in any way — the lighter the better. With your arms loosely at your sides, palms facing upwards, take a deep breath — deeply and slowly right from your chest and abdomen so that you expand your lungs fully. You should feel your abdomen swell and your diaphragm lower. Hold it while you count to five and then exhale slowly, letting out all the air, and relax.

Your abdomen will sink as the air is released. Practise this several times to experience the feeling.

Now that you feel more relaxed get to know your body better by experimenting with different muscle groups, gently stretching and flexing them, one at a time. Feel the stretch and become more aware of these muscles. Or, working downwards from the head, try relaxing different areas of the body in slow motion. First relax your facial muscles so that they feel free of tension or any taut, tight sensations, then your neck, your shoulders, your chest, arms, abdomen, hips, legs and feet. Do this gradually and slowly and when your whole body feels relaxed, try to wipe your mind free of conflicting thoughts and emotions. Either make it go blank or concentrate on one object or thought to the exclusion of all others. After 10 minutes, start regaining control of your body upwards from your feet to your head, and then stretch out as far as you can go, feet in one direction and arms in the other so that you extend your spine.

For some more advanced controlled breathing techniques try the following suggestions and practise them regularly, preferably out-of-doors or in front of an open window to get plenty of fresh air.

1 This exercise will help relieve tension and relax you. Standing up straight with your arms hanging loosely at your sides, slowly inhale through your nose. Hold for 5-6 seconds and then exhale slowly through your mouth. Repeat five times. Now when you inhale through your nose try lifting your shoulders and clenching your fists as you rise up on tiptoe. Keep holding your breath as you tense your body hard and then slowly lower your heels to the floor, relax your shoulders, open your fists and exhale slowly. Relax and repeat five times.

2 Sit cross-legged on the floor, with your back straight and your arms held behind you. Slowly breathe in deeply through your nose and rotate your head very slowly forwards and then round over your right shoulder and back round over your left shoulder to the front to form a complete circle. Slowly exhale and then repeat in the opposite direction. Do this three times in each direction and then relax. These head rolls are very relaxing.

3 Sitting cross-legged with your back held straight, close your left nostril with your left forefinger. Inhale deeply through the right and count slowly to 4. Now block the right nostril too and count to 4. Open the left nostril and exhale slowly through it. Then inhale deeply and close it again with your forefinger. Count to 4 and exhale through the right. Repeat this exercise four or five times. If practised regularly it will help you to breathe more deeply and control your breathing more efficiently. It is a useful exercise for yoga.

4 Sitting in a chair with your back straight, exhale deeply through your mouth to empty your lungs. Now inhale very slowly through your nose, pushing out your chest and abdomen as you slowly raise your arms above your head. Hold them aloft to a count of 6, and then exhale slowly through your mouth, lowering your arms and relax. Repeat five times.

All these exercises will help you to develop greater lung capacity, and if practised regularly you will begin to feel more relaxed and healthy with increased energy. Not only will you feel fresher and less tired but you will look better too as your skin and hair both benefit from more oxygen flowing to the cells and the more efficient removal of wastes from your system. For complete and total relaxation you can try the yoga corpse position for which you will need a long slanting hard board. Prop the board up against something so that the raised end is resting securely about 30cm/12in above ground level. Now lie down along the board with your head at the bottom and your feet at the top. Slowly relax your body from head to toe and maintain the position for 10-15 minutes. Then gradually regain control and relax.

Meditation

For many years, the exclusive realm of mystics and priests, meditation is now practised by a wide range of people including such varied groups as housewives, businessmen, teachers, scientists and lawyers. Since the Beatles' famous visit to the Maharishi Yogi in the 1960s, centres for transcendental meditation have been set up all over the world where you can go to learn the technique. However, other simpler and cheaper methods of meditation also exist which you can teach yourself at home. People who meditate regularly claim that it reduces stress and anxiety, increases their creativity, relieves

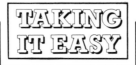

insomnia and encourages them to smoke and drink less. The benefits you receive from regular meditation, however, depend on what you are prepared to put into it. Scientists have established, by recording the physiological changes in people who are meditating, that certain beneficial changes do occur. For example, they discovered that the meditating body consumes less oxygen and its metabolic rate is actually lower than during sleep. Blood pressure is also lowered as are lactate levels in the blood. Breathing becomes slower and deeper, and even brain patterns become more relaxed. Thus although a state of mental alertness is maintained throughout, the body enters a phase of restfulness.

So meditation is not purely spiritual and contemplative; it can bring positive physical results for the body. Many people, of course, still ridicule the idea and regard it as a trendy, slightly frivolous thing to do, possibly because our culture and society tends to value action and material achievements rather than relaxation and inner comtemplation. There is nothing magical about the process of meditation — it is simply a means of relaxing your body and mind and relieving them of tension.

Sometimes the simpler meditative methods are the most effective. Before you rush out and enrol in a transcendental meditation course, practise sitting in a dimly lit room with your back straight and your legs crossed in front of you. Breathe in slowly and deeply until you establish a gentle rhythm. Now it is time to start repeating a *mantra*, either out loud or in your head. Basically, a mantra is a soothing sound, which is continually repeated to clear the mind of other thoughts and tension until the person enters a relaxed state. The sound gives you something to focus your mind on and the usual ones used are the vowel sounds: ah, eh, ih, oh and uh. Each of these sounds is related to the release of a physical or emotional sensation. Thus 'ah' diminishes anxiety; 'eh' relieves tension; 'ih' dissipates aggressive feelings; 'oh' brings release from physical pain; and 'uh' abates sexual tension. You can use any of these vowel sounds, or indeed any

calming sound or word which you like to repeat. Keep chanting your chosen mantra until all everyday thoughts disappear and your mind is left relaxed, pleasantly calm and free from tension. It is a curious feeling as you may appear almost detached in your new freedom.

Like anything else worth achieving, meditation takes practice and you cannot expect to feel wonderful and free the very first time you try. But persevere for 15 minutes every day and you will be able to clear your mind and free it from the constraints of your body. As a result you will feel more mentally alert with greater powers of concentration for tackling work and any problems that you may encounter. You will be less likely to feel tired and irritable as you discover the still centre of yourself and your very own inner tranquillity. This feeling of being at peace with yourself and your new self-knowledge will not only make you more confident and decisive but they will also improve the quality of your life. You will value these quiet moments of peace when you can escape from the pressures of modern-day living into the private world of your mind and discover your own creativity by sitting still and listening to your body. As life becomes more hectic and demanding, these quiet periods of inner comtemplation become more imperative than ever for us all.

Yoga

The word 'yoga' comes from the Sanscrit and literally means 'union', referring to the integration of mind, body and spirit. Thus it is an extension of meditation in that it seeks enlightenment through exercising and training the body as well as the mind. It is probably the best known and most popular form of meditation with thousands of devotees throughout the

The forwards stretch
1 *Stand up straight, feet together and arms extended above head. Exhale and slowly bend over from waist, keeping arms straight, palms together, as you lower them to floor.*
2 *Bring arms down to touch toes and push head and neck outwards and upwards. Keep your legs and back perfectly straight and hold the pose, breathing deeply. Repeat twice. This is a very relaxing stretch.*

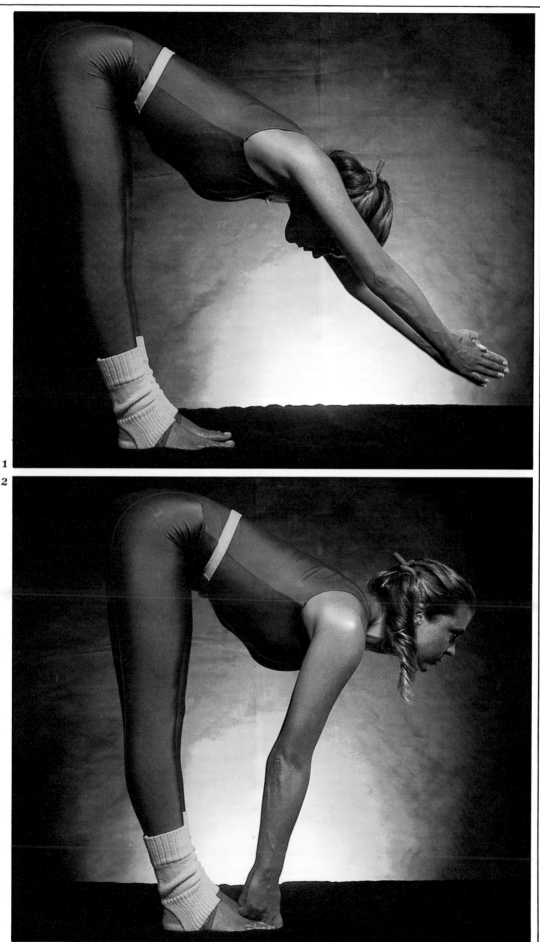

1
2

125

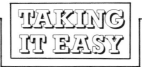

Western and Eastern worlds. Through a harmonious balancing and blending of mind and body, yoga can diminish tension, increase suppleness and bring peace of mind. Many people in stressful demanding occupations claim that just 15 to 20 minutes' yoga a day can help them cope better with daily pressures and the relief of tension.

According to yoga theory, we all have two different kinds of energy — male energy which is stimulating, dynamic and creative; and female energy which is restoring, gentle and calming. In most people these types of energy are unbalanced with the male sort having precedence over the female or vice versa. Yoga, however, strives to release them both and bring them into harmony. The yoga postures, or *asanas* as they are called, reflect this. Many of the strengthening asanas which are performed standing up release male energy, whereas more of the female-oriented asanas are performed lying down and are very relaxing. Yoga also tries to strike a balance between creativity, instinct and intellect by removing tension, releasing energy and encouraging creativity. It helps you to be more self-aware and to know your capabilities and limitations. Because it reduces stress and tension, it can help you to sleep better too as it leaves you feeling wonderfully calm and relaxed with a clear, uncluttered mind.

The energy released can be channelled into other areas of your life — your work, your leisure interests, sport and family. It is the perfect complement to aerobic exercise as it helps relax areas of your body and muscle groups that may be tightened or balanced disproportionately by running, cycling and other sports. And

because it gives you more suppleness and a wider range of movement, it helps you to perform better in other sports and exercise — thus you can run more efficiently, cycle faster and swim more powerfully. Increased suppleness and mobility make you less liable to get injured as most strains and muscle tears are caused when muscles get contracted and tight. Yoga stretches them slowly and safely, playing the muscles to the edge of their stretch and relaxing them.

As it helps to break down tension throughout your body, you feel freer and less inhibited physically, emotionally and intellectually. It is the perfect answer to hypertension which is becoming more

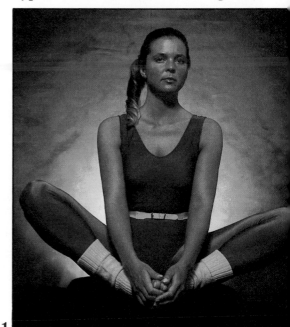

1

2

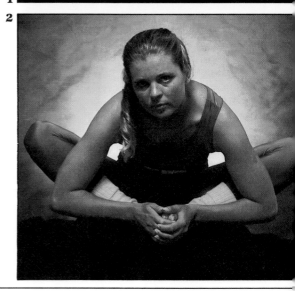

The butterfly
1 *Sit on floor with back straight, knees bent and the soles of your feet together, close to your body. Clasp your feet in your hands.*
2 *Slowly lean forwards over your body, towards the floor until your elbows are almost resting on the floor, your upper arms against your legs. Flutter your legs slowly up and down and feel the stretch in your inner thighs. Repeat the asana three times.*

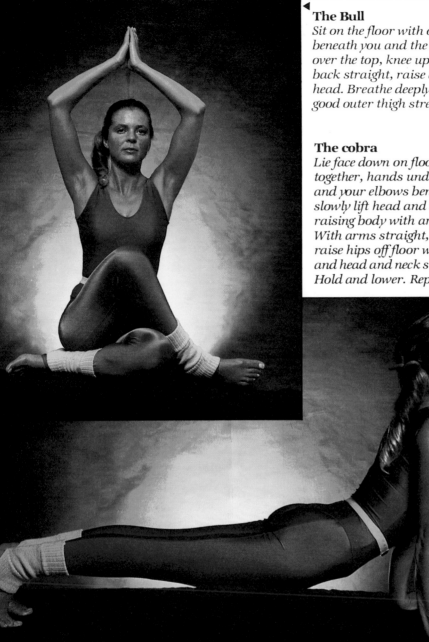

The Bull
Sit on the floor with one leg bent beneath you and the other bent over the top, knee up high. With back straight, raise arms above head. Breathe deeply. This is a good outer thigh stretch.

The cobra
Lie face down on floor with feet together, hands under shoulders and your elbows bent. Inhale and slowly lift head and shoulders, raising body with arm muscles. With arms straight, exhale and raise hips off floor with feet flexed and head and neck stretched back. Hold and lower. Repeat 4 times. ▼

prevalent in Western society — it is estimated that about one-third of people in the West now suffer from this. Breathing plays an important role in yoga, forming the essential balancing link between the mind and the body. To practise yoga, you must learn to breathe abdominally by inhaling right down to your pelvis (for specific exercises, turn back to page...). Breathing slowly and deeply in this way relaxes your muscles as well as your mind, aids circulation and blood flow to the brain and muscles, and has a calming, tranquillising effect.

You can join a class under the guidance of an instructor or practise yoga by yourself at home. Having said that, you may find it useful and stimulating when you are starting out to get some expert help or advice. Just put aside 20 minutes each day for deep breathing and some of the simple asanas, perhaps before you get up in the morning or when you go to bed at night — a time when you are feeling relaxed. Warm up before you start with a few gentle stretching exercises and some aerobics, such as running on the spot (see suggested exercises on page...). This will warm up your muscles and make them more flexible. The key to yoga is to perform the asanas slowly, gently and without straining. You should never bounce yourself into a given position as this will invoke the stretch reflex and is

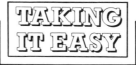
more likely to damage or shorten muscles that you want to extend and stretch. Each exercise should be performed slowly and thoughtfully, gently stretching until you reach the desired position. Hold it and concentrate on what you are doing but as soon as you start to feel any physical discomfort, slowly come out of the stretch and return to your original position. As you become more proficient and supple you will be able to hold the positions for longer. All the time concentrate on what you are doing and block out all other thoughts. You will be amazed at how calm and still you feel as you move slowly through each asana. Let your body go with the movement, not fight against it, and you will reap the benefits of relaxation. Listen to your body all the time and never overdo it. Yogis, of course, can go through the pain barrier but your body will be stiff at first and unused to the unfamiliar postures so learn to distinguish between discomfort and pain and gently withdraw from the asana as soon as it starts to hurt.

Afterwards, don't just jump up and get on with other things immediately. Instead, relax by lying on a flat surface with your lower back pressed into the floor and then very slowly allow your spine to return to its natural curve. Squeeze your shoulders together tightly and then relax them. Flex each foot, one at a time, to stretch out your leg muscles and then relax them. Allow your feet to fall outwards, your arms at your sides, palms facing upwards. When you are really relaxed concentrate on breathing deeply and rhythmically. Focus on your breath and clear your mind. Relax like this for 10 minutes and then gradually regain control of your body before getting up.

You should feel really relaxed with a clear, calm mind, but invigorated too with

The bow
Lie face down on floor and bend left leg, clasping your foot with your left hand. Now bend your right leg back and grip with right hand. Pulling on your feet and chest, slowly lift your chest and thighs off the floor. Stretch out your neck and head and slowly rock backwards and forwards, breathing deeply all the time as you feel the stretch.

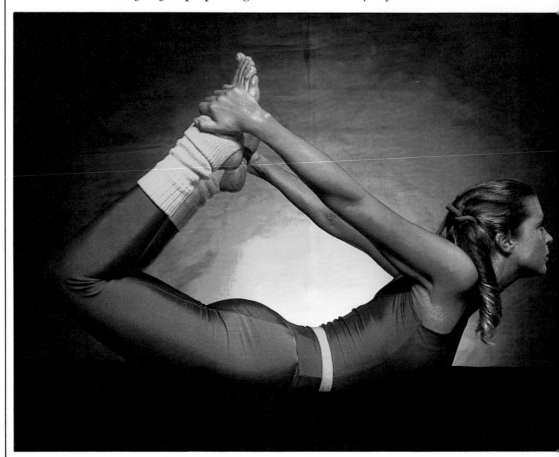

the energy to tackle other things. Try the asanas pictured here. They will all develop your strength and endurance as well as flexibility. Make them an indispensable part of your way of life.

Sleep

Sleep can be healing, restful and restorative and is vital for our health, both physically and psychologically. Nobody can stay fit and healthy without adequate sleep although the amount required varies from one person to another. Thus while most people consider that they need seven or eight hours sleep a night on average, others manage perfectly well on three or four hours. Usually the more stressful and demanding your day, the more sleep you need but this is highly individual. Certainly a lot of people probably sleep too much and would feel more energetic and vital if they slept less each night. Scientific studies have identified certain trends in sleeping habits and linked them to personality types. Thus short sleepers tend to be sociable, gregarious, active and conformist, whereas long sleepers are often introverted, creative and non-comformist.

While we sleep, our bodies are regenerated, cells are renewed and we are rested. However, it is not so simple as this for there are two kinds of sleep: slow-wave orthodox sleep and paradoxical dreaming sleep known as REM (rapid eye movement) sleep. While orthodox sleep restores the body, REM sleep maintains our emotional and mental stability. During the night you alternate between periods of orthodox and REM sleep, starting with orthodox sleep from the moment you drift off into blissful oblivion. The frequency of your brain-wave patterns slows down although their amplitude increases as you sink deeper into slumber. Your breathing becomes slower and more regular as your heartbeat decreases. Your blood pressure drops and, to an onlooker you appear relaxed and peaceful. However, as the night progresses short periods of REM sleep start to interrupt this serene sleep. When these

The camel
Kneel on floor, knees shoulder width apart, back straight and arms hanging at sides. Inhale and arch your spine, bending slowly backwards over your legs until you grasp your heels with your hands. Gradually move your stomach forwards and increase the stretch. Hold for a count of 5, breathing deeply. This improves your posture.

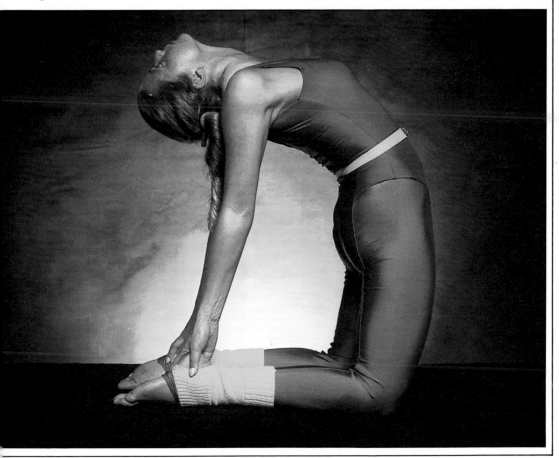

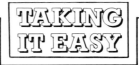

occur, your brain waves become irregular, and your temperature and blood pressure rise. As your heartbeat increases your breathing gets faster and more uneven. Your facial muscles and fingers may start to twitch and your eyes will move rapidly from side to side beneath your closed lids. All this activity probably lasts only from 10 to 20 minutes before you resume your peaceful sleep of before, but it recurs about once every one and a half hours on average throughout the night, culminating in a longer 30 minutes session just before you awake

During these periods of REM you dream, and thus REM sleep plays an important part in discharging tension and restoring calm and serenity to your nervous system. In experiments carried out on volunteers, scientists have attempted to discover more about the effects of REM sleep on our minds and health. When it is denied to sleepers and they are allowed only orthodox sleep they may become tense, even psychologically disturbed and depressed. When it is restored to them, they tend to enter these REM patterns for much longer as though to make up for what has been denied to them. Dreams are an outlet for removing tension and resolving inner conflicts so that we can wake refreshed. Some of our dreams may seem bizarre and inexplicable but this is because they are paradoxical and should not be taken too literally. We tend to dream in symbols and in allegory which conceal the dream's true meaning but at the same time they seek to communicate ideas and imagery between our conscious and subconscious minds. Dream examination is part of modern psychoanalysis of which Jung and Freud were pioneers when they attempted to penetrate dreams in depth. According to Jung, the dream is 'a little hidden door in the innermost and most secret recesses of the psyche'. There is no doubt that these dreaming REM periods of sleep are essential for restoring mental health and diminishing tension.

Drinking alcohol or taking barbiturates or tranquillisers can repress the REM dreaming phases and cause you to wake up feeling tired, irritable or depressed. If you take sleeping pills over a long period of time not only might they become physically and mentally addictive but they may also lead to increased tension and have lasting psychological effects. For women who cannot get to sleep, sleeping pills are a welcome means of relief initially but they may soon become an indispensable crutch. However, when you reach the stage that you believe that you cannot sleep without them it is probably not so much the chemical properties of the pill acting in conjunction with your nervous system that is sending you to sleep as the mere association in your mind between taking the pill and sleep. Try to analyse your attitude to sleep and any deeper reasons why you may not be sleeping before you succumb to sleeping pills. It might just be a temporary thing for a few nights when you sleep less and more intermittently, but getting only four or five hours of sleep a night does not necessarily label you as an insomniac. Perhaps this is all your body needs to renew itself. After a couple of bad nights you might worry so much about *not* getting to sleep that you sleep badly as a result. This is often self-induced and does not reflect a physical or emotional inability to sleep.

Most people have sleeping difficulties when they are going through traumatic or worrying phases of their lives. The waking hours between going to bed and getting up in the morning are a particularly anxious and frequently lonely time when sleep seems to be denied to you. Deep breathing and relaxation techniques can help, of course, calming your mind, taking tension out of your body and preparing you for sleep and relaxation. Most chronic isomniacs have tendencies towards severe depression and mental illness so it is unlikely that you are one of these. Your bad sleeping habits may stem from something much simpler, such as taking stimulants before you go to bed — for example, strong coffee can keep some people awake. Or they may even be related to diet in a small minority of cases where deficiencies of vitamin E, zinc or calcium can be identified, all of which lead to muscular tension. And having a few drinks to calm your nerves and send you to sleep is not effective either. Even if alcohol sends you to sleep you will probably wake several times throughout the night as it tends to make you sleep lightly and destroys the deep-sleep REM phases.

So if you have sleeping problems, what are the best ways of getting to sleep without having recourse to drugs? First, it is important to establish a regular sleeping pattern. It does not matter when you sleep as long as you establish a routine which you associate with sleep in your mind. Try to go to bed at the same time each night so that your body clock finds its own rhythm. Don't go to bed early to get extra hours of sleep if you do not feel tired. Go to bed late if you do not generally feel sleepy until then. A hot milky drink or some herbal tea can help relax your body as can a lukewarm bath so that you feel warm and already rested when you go to bed. Some people find that reading a book helps to get them in the right mood for sleep, although if it is very exciting and thought-provoking you may be encouraged to read late into the night, unable to put it down, and this could interfere with your sleep too. A few

minutes' meditating or going through some of the yoga postures can help relax your body and mind ready for sleep.

Regular physical exercise has also been pinpointed as a cure for insomnia. People who run, cycle, swim or play sports at least three times a week are likely to sleep soundly and wake up refreshed. Try it and see if it works for you. Aerobic exercise can help release tension and encourage a sense of emotional well-being and creativity that will permeate your whole life, helping you to sleep better and more productively.

The plough
1 *Lie flat on your back on the floor with arms at your sides. Slowly raise your legs off the floor until they are extended straight up above you. Supporting your body with your hands, lower your legs over your head behind you until they touch the floor.*
2 *For more advanced plough, extend arms flat along the floor, palms upwards. Hold the stretch for about 10 minutes.*

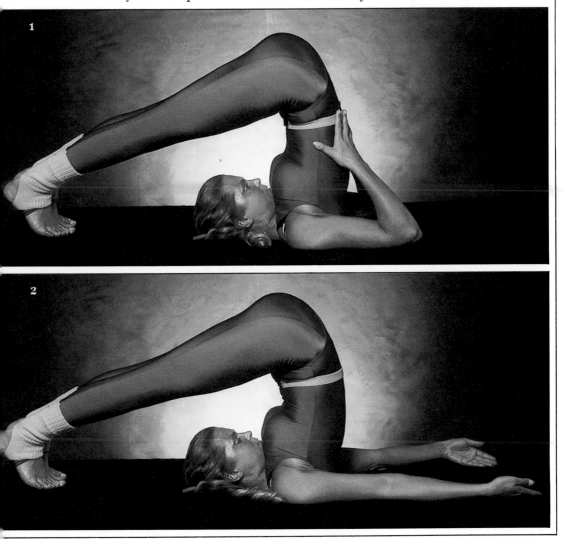

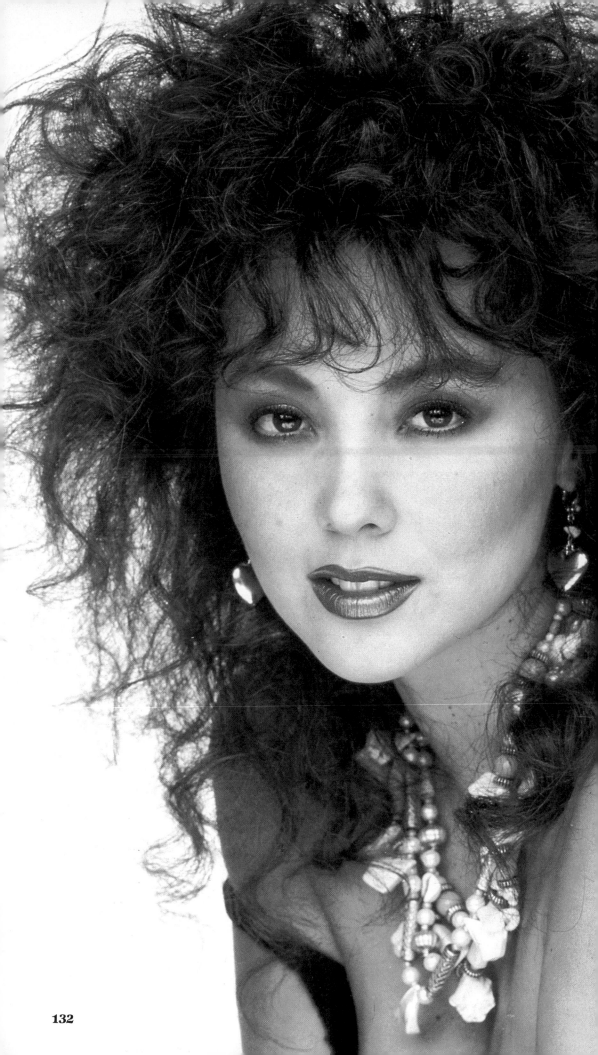

Marie Helvin

Top photographic model Marie Helvin believes in keeping fit and healthy. She thinks that people are now more aware of their bodies than ever before, and has evolved how own daily exercise regime to keep slim and trim for her demanding career. Every extra ounce shows up in the camera and so Marie spends 10 minutes every morning and another 10 minutes last thing at night on her mini-trampoline and exercise bike.

The beauty of her exercise routine is that it is simplicity itself and although she works abroad with her husband, photographer David Bailey, for six months every year, she can exercise wherever she goes with a jump-rope. She uses weights to strengthen her arms although, ''When I travel, I use bottles or beer cans instead.''

The modern trend of working-out to music does not appeal to her. She says, ''I don't like torture. I want to be gentle with my body.'' Instead, she prefers to exercise at home at her own pace, choosing exercises which she knows from experience do her good.

Eating healthily comes naturally to Marie and although she admits to loving peanut butter sandwiches and popcorn, she likes to eat wholefoods. She established her good eating habits as a child in Hawaii where she came from a large family. Her mother cooked only one big meal a day which they all had to eat. Now she still eats only when she is hungry and sticks to one main meal. She says, ''If it's at lunchtime, I just have salad or cheese and an apple in the evening. I have a large breakfast in winter, but just a piece of toast or something in summer.'' She prefers snacks and light meals to rich heavy dinners, does not like sugar and desserts preferring fresh fruit, and eats only fish, not meat.

She does not have to watch her weight too carefully to keep her naturally slim figure. ''I never had a weight problem,'' she says. ''Size 8 used to be the standard size for British models but now it's 10 which is much better for me. I used to weigh less but now I'm up to 125lb,'' which is perfect for her 5ft 9in.

Marie has taken multi-vitamin tablets every day since she was a child thanks to her father, a health and fitness fanatic. She also takes additional doses of vitamins A, C and E which help to keep her skin looking so fresh and beautiful. But although it looks perfect, Marie says that her skin is really quite dry. She cleanses it only once a day. ''I use rose water on it in the mornings before I moisturise and make-up. At night, I rub in natural oil, sunflower, safflower or apricot kernel, and then cleanse with pure natural soap and water. I never use night creams as I think they clog up the pores so that your skin can't breathe.'' When her skin is dry in winter and needs extra moisture, she squeezes 10 capsules each of vitamins A and E into some ordinary cheap moisturising cream. She has used this skincare regime for years and has never gone in for special eye creams and expensive body lotions. Instead, she uses margarine on her elbows, knees and legs to keep the skin soft and smooth. ''I like everything as simple and easy as possible and if I'm stuck when I'm away from home I can always make something.''

Her strong, thick dark hair has natural body and is always in excellent condition. Marie says, ''I wash my hair every day in summer. I hate it when it feels dirty and heavy. Clean hair should feel so light that you're not even aware it's there. Its like being bald.'' In winter she washes her hair less often — twice a week.

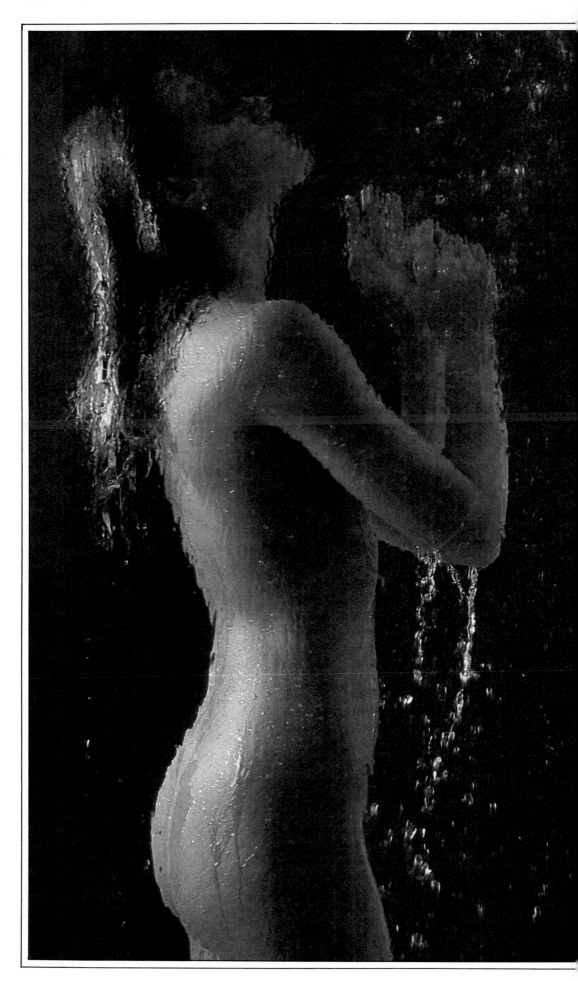

BODY MAINTENANCE

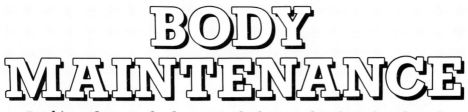

Looking after your body, particularly your skin, hair, hands and feet, is an important part of health and fitness. It is not just a form of self-indulgence as many people seem to think, but is necessary for your overall physical and mental well-being. Your body's shape and external condition reflect your internal health and even your emotions. The effects of stress, fatigue, poor diet and lack of exercise all manifest themselves outwardly in the way you look. Pallid, tired-looking skin, lank hair, brittle nails and stubborn patches of cellulite are usually the result of not looking after yourself — ignoring your body maybe or treating it carelessly. It needs a little pampering as well as general maintenance to keep it in first-class condition for your body is the physical expression of you and your feelings about yourself. If you neglect it, you are not being fair to yourself. It may be because you have negative feelings about your own potential and worth and are suffering from a lack of self-esteem.

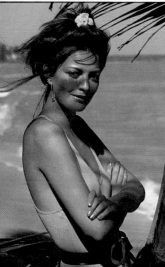

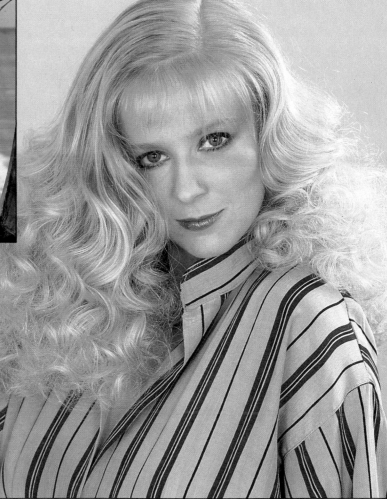

You have already learnt how your body is affected by what you eat and how you exercise and relax. Now you must understand how to keep it looking good and youthful by learning the arts of skin- and hair-care. Remember that it is a complex system of inter-related parts and sub-systems all working together and inter-acting with each other. If any part fails to work efficiently or if there is a weakness or imbalance in a sub-system or organ, it may affect other areas too and set up a chain reaction throughout the body.

The ups and downs of your lifestyle are also reflected in your body. Too many cigarettes or alcohol and your skin will suffer as well as your lungs and liver. Over-work, bad habits and the environment in which we live all take their toll and precipitate the ageing process within us. It's time we started taking care of ourselves, for feeling good is looking good and there are so many beauty spin-offs that you can enjoy — soft, glowing skin, glossy hair and a smooth, firm body full of vitality and energy. Start right now by looking at your skin.

Skincare

Weighing about 2.7kg/6lb and with a surface area of about 1.6 square metres/ 17 square feet, your skin is a good indicator of your general health, for it is affected from within by the food you eat, your level of stress, your balance of hormones and by physical illness. It is your largest organ and because it shows the tell-tale signs of age most clearly it is worth looking after. Good skin and a clear complexion are a woman's greatest beauty assets and a reflection of her inner health. But it is no good spending a fortune on expensive creams and cosmetics if you do not treat your skin from the inside as well as the outside. Good nutrition and regular exercise are also important, as we shall see.

Although the top layer of your skin consists of dead cells which are sloughing off all the time, underneath is living tissue — millions of cells nourished by an extensive network of capillaries through which the blood carries nutrients and oxygen. New cells are being formed in a continuous process and are pushed up towards the surface to replace the dead ones on top, although as you get older this complex process slows down and the top layer of epidermis cells is shed less easily. They become dry and coarse in appearance and consequently your skin looks older.

In addition to protecting and cushioning your body and forming a waterproof barrier on the outside, your skin seals in moisture, eliminates body waste into the atmosphere and keeps harmful bacteria and viruses at bay. It controls your body temperature and, through its network of sensory nerve endings, it transmits information about external stimuli to your brain. Thus it enables us to feel things, to experience painful and pleasant sensations and enjoy physical relations with other people.

To keep your skin looking radiant and healthy, you must learn to look after it properly. Good skincraft is not difficult nor is it time-consuming. It consists of feeding your skin the right nutrients, sealing in its natural moisture, keeping pores unclogged and free from toxic matter and pollutants, and protecting it from the damaging, ageing effects of the sun. However, some factors are beyond your control and these were determined even before you were born and are part of your genetic inheritance. They include your vulnerability to sunburn, the number of sebaceous glands and blood vessels in your skin and whether it is destined to be naturally oily, dry or normal. Try as you may, you cannot change these things and you must adapt your skincare routine and products to meet your skin's special requirements.

Whatever your skin type, skin consists of three layers: the outer epidermis (or stratum corneum); the underlying dermis; and, deepest of all, the hypodermis, or subcutaneous layer of fatty tissue and muscle. Each layer has its own specific functions and all three are closely inter-related.

The epidermis consists of a layer of flattened overlapping horny cells which are forever being shed and replaced from below. It takes three weeks for a new skin cell, formed in the underlying dermis, to travel to the outer epidermis and dry out, die and be shed. Your skin looks smooth and fresh when the cells lie flat against

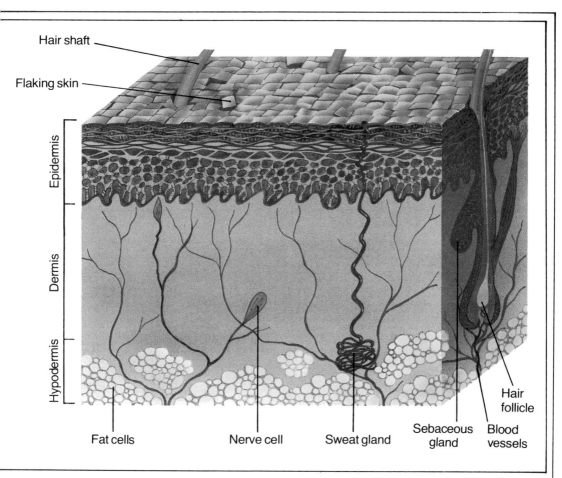

Hair shaft

Flaking skin

Epidermis

Dermis

Hypodermis

Fat cells

Nerve cell

Sweat gland

Sebaceous gland

Hair follicle

Blood vessels

each other but it will appear flaky and dry if their edges curl up. The epidermis is protected by a naturally acid mantle which deters bacteria and pollutants. This acidity is referred to as the pH factor of your skin and it usually lies in the range of 4·5 to 5·5. Alkaline cleansers and soaps can disturb the delicate balance of natural acidity and may cause spots and other skin problems.

The dermis contains the sebaceous oil glands, sweat glands, hair follicles, blood vessels, nerve centres, pigmentation cells and the *living* skin cells. It is also a reservoir of essential moisture for keeping skin soft and smooth. This is the working level of your skin where all the essential functions and processes are carried out and the blood vessels supply oxygen, protein, vitamins and minerals. Its connective network of tough collagen fibres gives your skin strength and firmness. Scientists have now discovered that these fibres, made up of protein and elastin, have to be supple to keep skin looking smooth and elastic. If they bunch up, or 'cross-link', your skin will start to sag and become wrinkled and lined with age. Cigarette smoking, alcohol, high lead

This cross-section through the skin shows its three layers: the epidermis, dermis and hypodermis. The skin you see is, in fact, the dead skin cells on the surface of the epidermis which are continually sloughing off and being replaced by new ones.

and aluminium levels in the body, illness and too much sun can all activate the cross-linking process in your skin and age it, as can deficiencies in vitamin C and zinc. Anti-oxidants, which discourage cross-linking by preventing the chemical bonds forming between the proteins, lipids and fats in your skin, include zinc, selenium, and vitamins A, B, C and E. You should make sure that you get plenty of these in your diet or take special supplements as they can slow down the ageing process and help protect your skin.

The hypodermis is made up of layers of subcutaneous fatty tissue and muscles which pad and insulate the body, giving skin its support and contour. Regular exercise plays an important role in maintaining the firmness, strength and elasticity of the muscles. If they become weak and sag, you skin will also sag and will lose its natural firmness.

The enemies of good skin

Healthy skin has many enemies, ranging from natural ones like over-exposure to the sun and cold weather, to unnatural ones which are directly related to our modern lifestyle and environment such as pollution and cigarette smoking. They are all potentially dangerous and ageing as they may promote cross-linking, coarse textured skin, an uneven blotchy complexion, blocked pores, skin irritations, and even cancer in the case of the sun.

When you smoke, the nicotine in the cigarette constricts tiny blood vessels in your skin, preventing blood being supplied to the cells and interfering with the removal of waste products. Efficient blood supply is vital for maintaining healthy skin and stopping pores getting blocked by waste materials. Many smokers suffer from premature wrinkling around their eyes and an unnatural pallor.

Even a little alcohol can affect your skin, disturbing its fluid balance and dilating the blood vessels, so that the cells are starved of oxygen. As the cells break down, tiny haemmorrhages occur, resulting in broken veins and a florid complexion. By the way, 'gin bags' are not a myth — they really can be caused by too much booze which softens the delicate tissue under the eyes.

Dirt and grime, dust, detergents and car fumes all affect our skin and may irritate it sometimes. Living in a city or beside a busy main road call for special skincare and thorough cleansing to remove deep-down impurities that may block pores. Some people are allergic to certain cosmetics and hair dyes which contain chemicals, colouring agents and preservatives. If you have delicate, sensitive skin, choose hypo-allergenic cosmetics, mild shampoos made from natural ingredients and unscented soaps. There are special ranges available which should not harm your skin.

Sun and climate

The quickest way to age and damage your skin irreparably is to spend a great deal of time in the sun. Everybody wants to have a lovely golden tan and to look glamorous and young but look closely at the skin of someone who has spent many summers in the hot sunshine and you will see that it looks dry and lined and starts to resemble old leather. Fair skinned sun worshippers are particularly at risk as they have little in-built protection against the sun's harmful radiation. If you spend only a couple of weeks' holiday a year sun-bathing there is little danger, but if you live in a hot sunny climate you should limit your sun-bathing and protect your skin with sun blocks or filters. Skin cancer is becoming increasingly common in the United States and Australia where people spend a lot of their leisure time out in the hot sunshine. For information on tanning safely see page 153. Tanning treatments are now available in most beauty salons and health clubs and many homes have their own mini sun lamps, but these are also dangerous if used regularly and will damage your skin's natural texture and moisture.

The climate and temperature can affect your skin too. Skin colour has evolved as a reponse to its natural climate, so most fair skinned people who live in colder regions cannot take as much sun as darker-skinned people from warmer climates who have more protective skin pigment. Cold weather and strong winds dry your skin as they accelerate its natural moisture loss. Intense heat, on the other hand, can damage small blood vessels in your skin as happens when you sit too close to a fire on cold winter evenings. Another winter hazard is poor circulation and this is the time of year when your skin may lose its healthy glow and look pale and dull. The best cure is exercise — brisk walking, jogging or working-out in the gym will all activate circulation and make your heart beat faster to pump more blood to starving skin tissues. It is also a good way of getting rid of impurities and waste products out of your system as it opens pores and encourages perspiration. Your skin will tingle and look pink and glowing afterwards. A less energetic way to promote circulation is to treat yourself to a herbal steam infusion. Just put some rosemary, thyme, or camomile in a large basin and

Although the current fashion is to have a natural glowing tan, the sun can be very damaging to skin so protect it always.

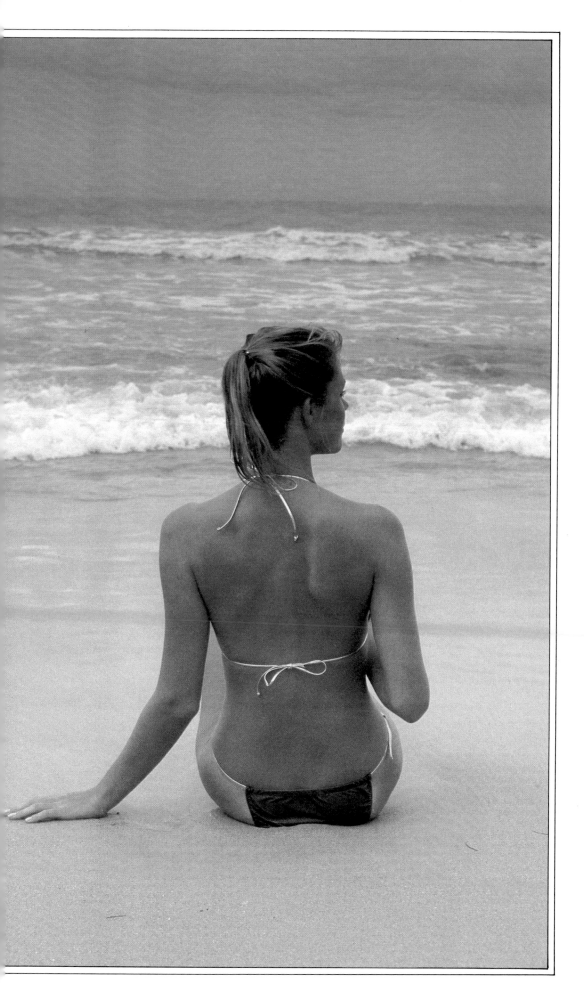

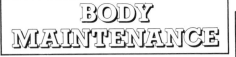

fill it near to the brim with boiling water. Cover your head with a towel, lean over the bowl and steam your face gently for 10 minutes. The steam will open clogged pores and draw out dirt and grease.

Diet and your skin

Poor diet is another enemy of good skin. Too many junk and convenience foods, fats and sugars all contribute towards problem, oily, coarse and sallow skins. Bear in mind when you eat your next chocolate bar or packet of French fries that your skin is a reflection of what you eat. It needs good food which is rich in nutrients to nourish it, keep it smooth and soft and aid circulation. Therefore it follows that the better your diet the clearer your skin. If you follow the guidelines for healthy eating set down in chapter 1 (see page 6) you cannot go far wrong. A diet that is high in fresh fruit, vegetables, salad stuffs and whole grain cereals with some protein and fatty acids and plenty of fibre will benefit your skin as well as your health. High-fibre foods and several glasses of mineral water per day will help eliminate waste products from your system which are often related to poor circulation and the build-up of cellulite. Include some protein in your daily diet (about 40-50g of fish or poultry or vegetable protein is sufficient) for cellular metabolism and the formation of healthy supportive collagen.

Cereals, fruit, vegetables and low-fat dairy foods will provide essential vitamins and minerals for feeding your skin. Vitamin A can prevent skin becoming dry and scaly. Good sources are shredded or chopped raw carrot in salads, and green vegetables (such as spinach, watercress and parsley), peppers and beans, apricots, peaches, eggs, skimmed milk and fish oils. The B-complex vitamins are also important for good skin-care and it appears that people who are deficient in these are particularly vulnerable to skin problems. Whole grains, liver, brewers yeast, beans and pulses, molasses and wholewheat bread will provide your nutritional requirements and help keep skin healthy with good circulation and efficient removal of waste products. Vitamin E has been hailed in recent years as the new miracle worker for tired ageing skin and many people swear by its anti-oxidant properties for it can prevent polyunsaturated fats being oxidised in the body and accumulating in the skin tissues. It also combats the toxic 'free radicals' in the skin often formed by the sun's powerful radiation. You can take vitamin E as a supplement, or sprinkle some wheat germ on your breakfast cereal. Many green vegetables, eggs, sunflower and safflower oils are also good sources. Vitamin C, or ascorbic acid, is found in citrus fruits, green vegetables, berry fruits, tomatoes and bean sprouts. It protects collagen fibres and keeps them strong and elastic to make your skin look youthful and healthy. Taken with zinc, it can help prevent wrinkles, sagging skin and stretch marks. Minerals, especially zinc, sulphur, iodine and selenium, also play a part in the maintenance of good skin. Mineral water and a well-balanced healthy diet should supply your body's needs.

Hormones and your skin

Hormonal imbalances can also affect the quality of your skin. This is especially noticeable at puberty when skin often looks coarse and oily due to over-stimulated sebaceous glands, and many teenagers suffer from pimples and acne. We all have a mixture of male and female hormones but occurring in varying proportions. Oestrogen and progesterone, the female hormones, make our skin look finer, more delicate and less oily, whereas androgen, the male hormone, is responsible for oily, coarse textured skin. Thus women tend to suffer more from dry skin as they get older but taking oestrogen can bring about an improvement as many women who take the contraceptive pill have found. During pregnancy your skin changes, usually becoming clearer and finer with a radiant pink bloom as hormonal changes take place within your body. You may also have noticed that it looks different at various stages of your menstrual cycle, being more oily and prone to spots and pimples immediately before and during a period.

Basic skincare

The way in which you care for your skin depends on your skin type — whether it is normal, oily or dry, or a combination of these. The basic characteristics of your skin, its colour and texture, are hereditary

Skin Chart Use this chart to work out your personal skin type and how to treat it.

Skin type	Characteristics	Skincare	Ageing	Exercise	Pollution
Dry sensitive skin	Sensitive skin which is dry and flakes easily. Burns easily and may be freckled. May have broken capillaries and fine lines.	Use a gentle cleanser and moisturise well. Use alcohol-free toner.	Moisturise thoroughly to stop skin drying out and ageing.	Exercise keeps skin smooth and with less lines.	Dries and dehydrates skin even further. Cleanse frequently and moisturise well to replace water loss.
Oily skin	Sallow and shiny with enlarged pores and prone to blemishes and blackheads, also spots. May look coarse. Tans very easily without burning.	Cleanse with gentle soap and use oil-absorbing moisturiser. Exfoliate often and use masks to control oil.	Ages well as does not dry out fast. Not so prone to lines and wrinkles.	Remove make-up before exercising, cleanse afterwards. Keep hair off face.	May increase oiliness so cleanse with gentle soap and toner and then moisturise with water-in-oil products.
Normal balanced skin	Smooth, supple skin which retains moisture and elasticity without shine or enlarged pores. Few blemishes or lines. Tans slowly.	Cleanse and tone each day and use moisturiser.	Moisturise more frequently as you get older to help prevent lines and wrinkles.	Cleanse after exercise. Skin will glow with healthy.	Protect skin with moisturising barrier, using more in windy cold weather. Cleanse well morning and night.

and there is little you can do about these, but the way you eat, exercise and treat your skin influence its general condition and combat excessive oiliness or dryness and delay the ageing process. To work out your skin type, cleanse thoroughly to remove all traces of make-up. After 30 minutes or so, examine your skin closely in a mirror and blot it with a clean tissue. If it is shiny with open pores and the tissue is greasy, your skin is oily. If, on the other hand, it looks matt with a soft bloom and not a trace of oiliness or dryness, then you are one of the fortunate few who has normal, balanced skin. However, it is quite likely that you do not fall completely into any one of these categories. Most people have a combination skin, that is, they have a central oily panel running down from the forehead through the nose to the chin, and dry or normal cheeks at the sides. If your skin is like this, you may have to treat specific areas in different ways and adapt you skincare routine accordingly.

Normal balanced skin is smooth, moist and unblemished but very rare. It is an ideal state of affairs in which moisture, acidity and oil are perfectly balanced. Although it does not shine or flake and is less prone to lines and wrinkles than dry

This helpful skin chart will tell you at a glance how to care for and protect your skin against ageing and environmental pollution.

skin, it still needs careful cleansing and moisturising to keep it looking good, and an adequate healthy diet to feed it the nutrients it needs to stay in top condition.

Dry sensitive skin tends to flake easily, to be super-sensitive to sun and often looks fine and taut. Because it is so sensitive, it lines and wrinkles easily and may have broken tiny veins and a reddish tone. It may be allergic also to some harsh cosmetics and skincare products and break out in rashes and irritations. Dry skin needs more loving care than any other skin type to seal in its natural moisture and prevent it becoming very dry and lined as it ages easily. Dry atmospheres, and strong winds all dry it out even more and therefore it needs regular moisturising to keep it smooth and supple.

Oily skin can be a disadvantage or a blessing in disguise, for although it is prone to blemishes and blackheads, it does improve as you grow older and ages more slowly than dry or normal skin. It becomes oily when the oil glands produce too much sebum, causing it to appear shiny with open pores. Drying the skin out with harsh soaps and astringents may dry it so much that the glands are stimulated into producing yet more oil to compensate for the loss of natural oils. The new thinking on caring for oily skin emphasises gentler and more thorough cleansing with special pH balanced products to keep the skin really clean and retain its naturally acid protective mantle.

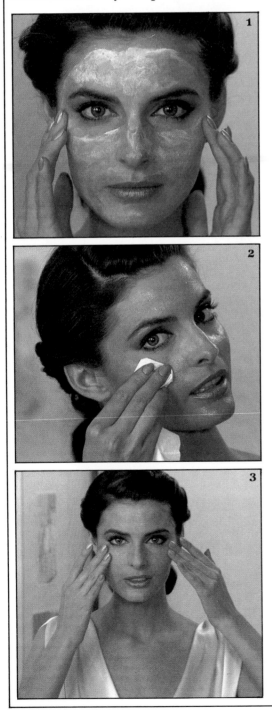

Most skincare regimes consists of three basic procedures: cleansing, freshening and moisturising. They may sound complicated and time-consuming but 10 minutes a day, night and morning, will help keep your skin smooth, fresh and young so it is worth making it an indispensable part of your daily routine when you get up in the morning and before you go to bed at night. It is the *only* way to ensure good healthy skin. Other useful skincare methods include exfoliating, conditioning face masks and facial saunas. You can treat yourself to these special treatments once every week or fortnight, depending on your skin type. They need not be expensive — many are prepared with natural ingredients from your refrigerator or vegetable rack — and they can be carried out at home in some free time when you feel like relaxing and pampering yourself without a visit to a costly beauty salon. But let's look first at the basic skincare routine for your face. We will consider looking after your body in the sections on bathing and caring for feet and hands on pages 148 and 150.

Cleansing twice a day will keep your skin healthy, clean and fresh and will help remove dead cells from its surface. Because your skin is basically an organ of elimination through which waste materials are removed from your body, it is important to keep pores open and free from blockages. Blocked pores lead to spots, pimples and skin problems, so make sure that your cleansing removes any grime, dirt, grease, stale make-up and other impurities. When it comes to which sort of cleanser to use for this task, there are many different products and opinions as to which are best. Some people swear

You should make this easy skincare routine part of your everyday life to ensure young-looking, smooth skin for years to come.
1 Cleanse thoroughly to remove stale make-up, dirt and grease. Wash off with warm water or remove with tissues.
2 Tone your clean skin with a mild freshener to strip away any remaining make-up and leave skin really squeaky clean.
3 Moisturise to add or seal in your skin's natural moisture and keep it soft and smooth and plumped-out.

by good old-fashioned soap and water, whereas others prefer cleansing milks, creams, oils and lotions. There is no doubt that a good lathering with a mild soap does make your skin feel really squeaky clean afterwards, but 'mild' is the operative word here. Most ordinary household brands of soap are highly alkaline and often contain harsh detergents which will strip away your skin's natural acidity and moisture, making oily skin even oilier through over-stimulation of the sebaceous glands, and dry skin even dryer. If you like to use soap for cleansing, then choose one of the specially formulated detergent-free pH balanced soaps which are now made by many beauty houses. They will effectively dissolve dirt and grease without damaging the skin's natural acidity and moisture. Foaming cleansers can also be used with water and work on the same principle.

If you dislike the soap-and-water method, you may prefer to use one of the specially formulated creams, milks, or lotions. Many of these work even deeper than soap to leave your skin really clean, although it may not feel as fresh. Whichever method you choose, it is important to cleanse twice every day and make it an unbreakable and enjoyable habit — as natural as cleaning your teeth!

Freshening, or toning, removes any traces of dirt, grease or make-up that your cleanser failed to strip away. It refreshes and stimulates your skin, leaving it smooth and glowing. Harsh astringents are a thing of the past, and gentler, alcohol-free fresheners are best for all skin types. If you prefer to use natural products, try witch hazel, cucumber or lemon tonics (specially good for oily skin) or just a mixture of cider vinegar and water. Apply with a cotton wool pad and then pat dry with a tissue.

Moisturising is the most important feature of skincare if you are to keep skin smooth, supple and free from lines and premature wrinkles. The function of a good moisturiser is to protect the skin's natural moisture and prevent its unnecessary loss. In effect, it forms a protective barrier between your skin and the environment, guarding against dehydration, reducing evaporation from the cells and keeping out dirt and pollution. It can also restore moisture to dry, flaky skin and plump it out so that it looks smoother and younger, with a softer texture. Moisturising becomes more important as you grow older and your skin's natural reserves of moisture gradually diminish. Some of the new moisturising products which contain soluble collagen and amino acids can penetrate really deeply to help cell renewal and replacement and speed up the normal biological processes within your skin to keep it looking younger.

Oil-in-water emulsions are quite effective as they attract any moisture in the air to supplement your skin's natural supply. Water-in-oil moisturisers prevent moisture already in your skin evaporating into the atmosphere by forming a protective film on the surface. They are the best products for dry, sensitive and normal skins to prevent excessive moisture loss through daily transpiration. They can be used safely on oily skin also as they do not stimulate the sebaceous glands to produce more oil.

Always moisturise in the morning after cleansing and freshening before applying make-up, and again in the evening before you go to bed. This will help protect your skin against environmental pollution, bacteria, and the drying effects of sun and wind, central heating and air-conditioning. Installing a humidifier in your home or office can help reduce natural moisture loss from the atmosphere and may pay dividends where your skin is concerned.

Special treatment creams that contain amino acids and soluble collagen are ideal for dry and ageing skins. Regular daily treatments can often effect good results and make skin appear younger, smoother and softer to the touch in a matter of weeks.

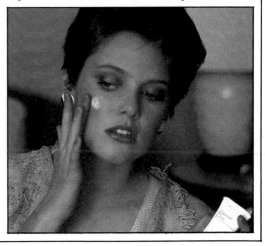

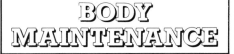

Special treatments are additional to your normal daily skincare routine and are sometimes necessary to condition and revive tired-looking skin, stimulate cell growth and metabolism, and cleanse really deeply to draw out stubborn waste and impurities that ordinary cleansing fails to remove. You can choose between the specially formulated masks, exfoliators and commercially produced facial saunas, and more natural products using fruit, vegetables, eggs, yoghurt, whole grain cereals and other ingredients. The naturally high enzyme content of many fresh fruits and vegetables can stimulate and beautify your skin but they must be used immediately after cutting or preparing if they are to be effective, as they oxidise very quickly after coming into contact with the atmosphere. The best time to treat your skin is after a bath or some vigorous exercise when your circulation has been stimulated and the pores are open and penetrable.

Face masks are great for revitalising skin and giving it a refreshing, toning deep cleanse which removes dirt, grease and toxic waste deep down in the pores. There are several types, including the ones you peel off and others that you rinse off with water. Most of them set on your face to a hard mask, stretching and tightening the skin underneath so that it feels really taut. This is not uncomfortable but merely soothing. Many are based on clay, earth or seaweed, and these are excellent for oily skins. The gentler, peel-off masks which harden like transparent skin across your face are more suitable for dry and normal skins. If you have a sensitive skin with broken veins, avoid the clay masks as they can cause further damage. Always remember to apply the mask to your neck as well as your face and remove it thoroughly after the allotted time taken for it to be effective. You will see that your skin looks plumper, pinker and glowing after the mask is removed. These effects

A special facial at a beauty salon can improve the texture and appearance of your skin, making it look fresher and more radiant. The skin is cleansed really deeply, often with steam or ozone, and then massaged and moisturised. It is an excellent treatment for dry and problem skins.

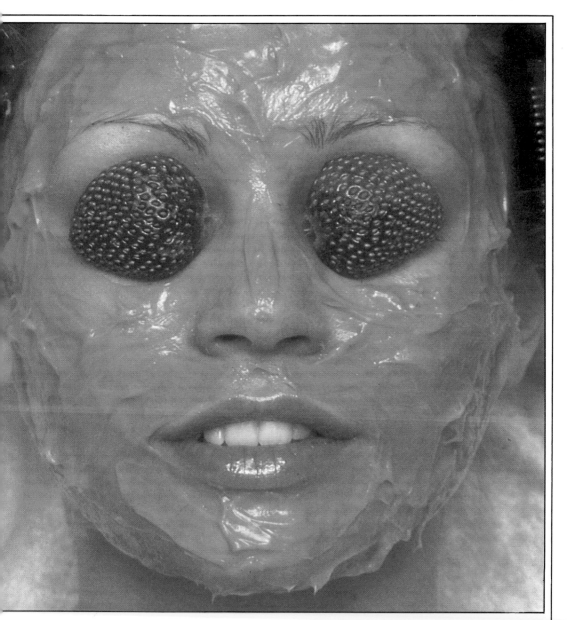

may be temporary or longer-lasting, depending on the product and your skin-type, but there is no doubt that oily skins will benefit from this treatment if it is used once or twice a week, and on other skins once every fortnight.

If you prefer to use natural products, the following suggestions are all effective, and you can experiment to discover which is best for your skin.

1 Mash an avocado and mix with live natural yoghurt. Smoothe over the face and neck and leave for 20 to 30 minutes before rinsing off.

2 Beat a few drops of lemon juice into an egg white and cover your face with this. Leave for 20 minutes and rinse off.

3 Crush a few strawberries and mix with a little oatmeal and some live yoghurt. Spread lightly over the face and neck. Leave for 30 minutes and rinse off.

A strawberry yoghurt face mask will look bizarre but it will leave your skin feeling soft and refreshed. You can mix it yourself and add a little oatmeal if wished (see suggestion 3 below). Alternatively, try out one of the other interesting ideas outlined here.

4 Mix some brewer's yeast with live natural yoghurt. Leave for 20 minutes and then rinse off with warm water.

All these masks stimulate and tone the skin, and the avocado mask is especially good for moisturising and softening.

Exfoliating is the term used for removing the dead cells and waste matter on the surface of the skin. This deep cleansing method stimulates the growth and reproduction of new cells in the underlying dermis and refines the skin so that it looks brighter, healthier and more translucent afterwards. After exfoliation, it is easier to moisturise your skin as the barrier of dead cells, make-up and toxic waste that clogs and blocks pores has been removed. Most exfoliating creams, gels and lotions contain suspended granules which are mildly abrasive and slough off the top layer of old dead cells, Exfoliation is not usually necessary for young skins but you should practise it once a week from your late twenties/early thirties onwards to stimulate new cell growth. Whereas it takes only 28 days for a new skin cell to travel from the dermis to the epidermis when you are a teenager, this time increases to at least 35 days in middle age and so exfoliation becomes more imperative than ever before to ensure that new cells come to the surface.

Facial saunas open up blocked pores and cleanse the skin of dirt, grease and impurities. If you live or work in a busy city and encounter car fumes, dirty air and pollution, then treat yourself to a weekly facial sauna. You need not buy a special machine — just place some fresh herbs in a basin, top up with boiling water, cover your head with a towel and, leaning over the water, gently steam your face for 10 minutes. The steam will soften your skin and improve general circulation. Afterwards, it will feel really fresh and clean, pink and glowing. However, facial saunas are not for people with highly delicate, sensitive skin or broken veins. Use another cleansing method if you fall into this category. They are an excellent way to tone oily skin and very soothing. Use sage, comfrey or fennel for dry skins; mint, camomile, nettle or rosemary for oily skins; and lavender, rose petal, elder-flower and peppermint for normal skins.

Problem skins

Although we all want clear, unblemished skin, not many of us achieve this ideal and most of us are beset by problems and blemishes at some time or another, whether it's acne in our youth or lines and wrinkles as we grow older. Even with a good diet, plenty of exercise and fresh air, adequate cleansing and hypoallergenic cosmetics, you can still get skin problems ranging from the odd pimple to broken veins, acne or even allergies and skin

rashes. Here is a run-down of the common problems and some advice on how to treat yourself and when to seek professional help.

Acne is usually a teenage problem which is associated with the onset of puberty and the hormonal changes in the body during this time. However, it does not always go away as you grow older, and many adults too are plagued by this distressing problem. Basically, it occurs when the male and female hormones are imbalanced and do not regulate the output of oil from the sebaceous glands, which secrete too much oil and become infected. The pores get blocked and the infection spreads.

In treating acne, many doctors and dermatologists tend to overlook the nutritional aspect. A healthy diet based on fresh wholefoods will help clear it up or, at least, make it a little better. If you suffer from acne, then change your eating habits as suggested in chapter 1 (see page 6). Eliminate sugary soft drinks, cakes, desserts, chocolate, biscuits, white refined flour, fats and junk foods from your diet, and eat along the guidelines laid down, paying special attention to fresh fruit and vegetables as these are high in minerals and vitamins. You can try taking additional vitamin supplements of A, B3, B6 and C, as these are thought to be beneficial in treating acne.

Good skin hygiene and really deep cleansing are also important. Cleanse thoroughly twice daily with a mild pH balanced soap or cleanser — harsh astringents and alkaline products may aggravate the condition further. Some gentle medicated creams and lotions are available too, as are some special creams and ointments which are available only on a doctor's prescription. Some doctors prescribe antibiotics in mild doses to fight the bacteria and this treatment often produces good results, as can sunshine in small doses. However, ultraviolet rays appear to make the condition even worse in some people.

Even after acne has cleared up and the skin is functioning normally again, permanent scars often remain to spoil a clear complexion. You cannot attempt to remove these scars yourself. Most can be covered lightly with a good foundation and translucent powder. If you are worried about them, you should consult a qualified dermatologist or plastic surgeon as highly specialised treatments are the only means of removal. These include dermabrasion, chemical peeling and plastic surgery.

Spots and pimples have many causes: oil blockages in the pores of the skin; the erratic shedding of skin cells; and poor cleansing which does not remove waste and impurities effectively. Hormonal fluctuations may be responsible too, and thus most women find that spots tend to break out at a certain time of the menstrual cycle, notably just before a period. Deep cleansing and regular exfoliation can help control them and stimulate new cell growth to keep cell metabolism functioning smoothly. Do not wait until the spots appear to treat them — instead, practise a little preventive medicine and exfoliate before your period starts to stop them forming at all. A healthy diet with plenty of bottled mineral water to eliminate body wastes will also help. When pimples appear, keep the surrounding skin scrupulously clean and use a medicated lotion on the affected area until they clear up. Once the pus comes to the surface and is released, the spot will soon heal without leaving a scar.

Blackheads are usually the result of poor cleansing and they tend to form in the oily central panel on the forehead, around the nose, mouth and chin. When oil becomes trapped in the pores it may blacken through oxidation when exposed to the air, and a blackhead forms. It is not dirt trapped under the skin as many people mistakenly believe. Again, good cleansing, regular exfoliation and a weekly face mask will help prevent them. To remove blackheads, steam your face gently for 10 minutes over a bowl of hot water until the pores are open and receptive. With clean hands, gently squeeze the blackhead out by inserting pressure with the tips of your fingers on either side. Afterwards, dab the area lightly with an antiseptic lotion. If you prefer not to use your fingers, you can buy special gadgets for their removal from most drugstores.

Whiteheads are beads of trapped oil just below the surface of the skin. Unlike blackheads which are open to the air, whiteheads lie beneath the epidermal layer of dead cells and should not be squeezed or the oil may leak into the underlying dermis and set up an inflammation. Dab whiteheads regularly with a mild medicated lotion and eventually they should disappear.

Oily skin is reponsible for many other skin problems, especially pimples, whiteheads and blackheads. Poor diet, overactive sebaceous glands which produce too much oil, hormonal imbalances and vitamin B deficiency are among the known causes. Although it is a nuisance as the skin seems to shine through even the most carefully applied make-up and has a tendency to break out in spots, it does not dry and age as quickly as other skin types. Excessive oil production can be controlled through a diet that is low in fats and refined foods and high in fresh vegetables, fruit, liver and whole grains. Vitamin B supplements are also an excellent idea. Like dry skin, it is delicate and not as tough as its sometimes coarse appearance would have us believe, so treat it like fine porcelain with great care and do not be tempted to dry it out with harsh astringent lotions and masssive doses of ultraviolet light which will only activate the sebaceous glands still further. Use mild foaming cleansers and oil-in-water moisturisers.

Sensitive allergic skin is becoming common as the atmosphere becomes more polluted and an increasing number of people eat refined and convenience foods which have been treated with chemical additives. Synthetic fibres, household detergents and cleaners, fertilisers and insecticides also play their part in activating allergic reactions in some people's bodies, particularly in the skin, which may become red, sore and itchy. Your body will react to an allergen by making antibodies to fight it off, but these sometimes combine with the allergen to release histamines which result in an ugly skin rash. This is why antihistamines are often used to treat allergies. Some of the common substances and foods that are known to cause allergic reactions in many people are wheat, milk, food colourings and additives, some perfumes, perfumed cosmetics and soaps, deodorants, lanolin, household cleaners, ammonia and washing powders, especially of the biological sort. Although dairy foods, especially milk and cheese, are allergens for some people, most healthy wholefoods are safe to eat. If you suspect that you are allergic to a particular substance, then you can go to your doctor and ask to be tested, or you can keep a record of what you eat and the cleaners and cosmetics you use and try gradually eliminating the suspect ones until you discover what is causing your rash. This process of elimination may take time but you will be relieved to know the identity of the allergen so that you can avoid it in future. Sometimes after six months or so of not eating a specific food or using a certain cosmetic, it may be safe to gradually introduce it again without suffering any allergic reactions. Meanwhile, use hypoallergenic make-up and cleansers which are fragrance-free, and treat sore or itchy rashes with soothing calamine lotion and witch hazel.

Eczema and dermatitis are often caused by allergies, although stress and anxiety, hereditary factors and high levels of toxic minerals in the body, especially lead, may also be responsible. The most common skin disease of all, the term eczema is derived from a Greek word meaning to bubble or boil, and this aptly describes the inflamed skin and blisters which are characteristic of this skin disorder. Patch testing can be carried out by your doctor to discover the cause of allergic eczema. Many chemicals are irritants, especially household cleaners and detergents. Nail polish, nickel in jewellery, lanolin, rubber and some preservatives are also known causes. Although eczema looks unpleasant it is neither contagious nor infectious, and if you can discover what is causing your eczema then you can control it by avoiding that substance. Failing that, you will have to consult your doctor for a suitable treatment with drugs or creams. Use mild hypoallergenic cosmetics and cleansers and soothing emulsifying creams on dry, sore skin.

Broken veins always need professional treatment, usually sclerotherapy which involves injecting a chemical fluid into the vein. Although they are usually hereditary, they may also be caused by poor circulation and inactivity which causes the blood to be concentrated in specific areas rather than flowing normally through them. Poor diet, smoking and sunshine can make them worse, so you should ensure that you protect the affected areas with a good sunscreen, stop smoking and eat plenty of vitamins B and C and zinc which all improve circulation. Regular exercise may also help. They can be concealed by make-up.

Discoloured skin and brown pigmentation are also difficult to remove. They can occur at any age — from taking the contraceptive pill or during pregnancy during your youth, or as age-spots as you get older. Hormonal changes and sunbathing may also trigger off brown patches and spots on the skin. The usual means of removal are deep peeling and planing techniques or the use of liquid nitrogen or frozen carbon dioxide. These methods can be performed only by professionals and cannot be attempted yourself. Sometimes uneven pigmentation will eventually disappear but small patches can usually be disguised effectively by the clever use of make-up, especially on the face. Do not expose them to the sun or they will become even more prominent.

Bathing

Good skincare involves not only looking after your face but also caring for your body by regular bathing to keep skin fresh and smelling sweet. The stimulating, healing and relaxing properties of water have been recognised for many years since people first started to visit health spas and 'take the water' in eighteenth century Europe. However, you do not have to travel to a spa town or a bubbling mud pool to enjoy the benefits of water — bathing or showering at home can be therapeutic also, and there is nothing like it for feeling really clean and refreshed. To lie back in a warm bath at the end of a busy day is relaxing and soothing, whereas a brisk shower first thing in the morning wakes you up and stimulates your skin, leaving it glowing.

Choosing the right temperature for your bath or shower will determine whether the experience is exhilarating, revitalising or calming. Not many people nowadays go in for Spartan ice-cold dips but many of us tend to wallow in baths which are much too hot for us and even damaging. So follow the rough guide below when you are bathing.

Hot : 95° — 110°F/34° — 43°C
This temperature range is too high, especially if you have a weak heart or circulation problems. Far from being stimulating or even soothing, hot baths will leave you lacking in energy, and if taken regularly will eventually lead to a sagging bosom, slack, loose skin and muscles, and broken veins. They are also very drying on the skin.

Warm : 85° — 95°F/29° — 34°C
This temperature range is best for a relaxing, luxurious wallow in the bath or a warm shower. It will ease the aches and pains in tired muscles and is sensual and soothing at the end of a hard day.

Tepid : 75° — 85°F/24° — 29°C
This is the perfect bath or shower for cooling down and relaxing in hot weather. It encourages good circulation and revives and refreshes you.

Cold : 55° — 65°F/13° — 18°C
This temperature is more suitable for a quick bracing shower to stimulate your circulation rather than a soak in the bath tub. With a powerful jet of water trained on muscles, it will prove a good skin tonic and will certainly wake you up in the morning!

Here are some exercises for you to try out when you are sitting in the bath:
1 Sit upright, fingers and toes resting on the bottom, stomach held in tightly.
2 Now keeping your back straight, raise your legs. Hold for a count of 2, lower and repeat 10 times, always very slowly.
3 Sit up straight with your legs bent beneath you, your hands clasped behind your back on the floor of the bath. Raise your arms slowly. Hold for a count of 3. Lower. Repeat the exercise 10 times.
4 Lie back in the bath, one leg extended underwater and the other raised. Move it in a circle. Lower, and repeat with the other leg. Repeat 10 times on each leg.
5 Sit with soles of feet together, holding onto edge of bath. Lower knees downwards, hold for a count of 3. Repeat 10 times.
6 Sit with arms raised, legs extended. Raise and lower legs alternately 10 times, lifting your legs clear of the water.

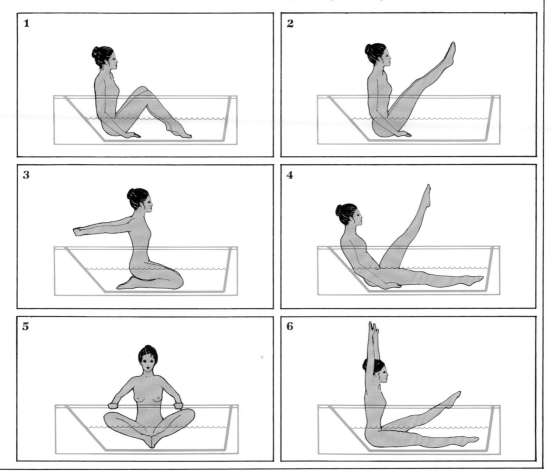

Bathing beauty

Bathing is more sensual and pleasurable in fragrant, scented water but you must know which foams, soaps and oils to use as some soften and beautify your skin while others are very drying. Always use a mild pH balanced soap which will not remove too much of your body's natural protective acidity, and do not use a soap at all if you add bath foam to the water. Most foams are quite drying so be sure to use a moisturising body oil on your skin after rubbing yourself dry with a towel. Oils of plant extractions are the best bathing beauty aid. Just a few drops of perfumed bath oil in the water will leave your skin feeling moist and smelling fragrant. Each plant oil has its own distinctive aroma and properties and your choice of oil will depend on your motivation for bathing. For example, lime blossom and lavender are both relaxing and encourage sleep, whereas pine and thyme are invigorating, bran is calming and softens the skin, and walnut oil is helpful in treating problem skin. Other fragrant oils include basil, rosemary, citron, jasmine, patchouli, rose and cardamom. They are all preferable to bath foams and detergent-based products which can irritate sensitive skin. Oils, on the other hand, will leave your skin moist and silky smooth.

The ancient Egyptians used to bathe in asses milk and you can follow their example by adding a cup of dried non-fat instant milk to the bath water. This helps soften dry skin. Mix in a few drops of aromatic oil to give it a lovely fragrance. A monthly salt bath will remove dead skin cells and flush out toxic waste in your body. Rub all over vigorously with coarse sea salt, avoiding sensitive areas. Then soak in a warm bath for half an hour (you can add salt to the bath water if wished). Afterwards you will feel fresh and invigorated and your skin will be pleasantly tingly. Rub yourself dry, wrap up warmly and relax for 15 minutes.

Another way of making bath water smell lovely is to sew some fresh herbs or dried flowers inside a thin muslin or cheesecloth bag and immerse it in the bath. Try using thyme, basil, rosemary, elderflowers, camomile and lavender. And instead of lying back in your scented bath and just going limp, work on patches of dead and rough skin on your feet, knees, elbows and thighs with a nail brush or loofah. A friction or a hemp glove is a good investment as it sloughs off dead cells and boosts circulation. One of the specialised massage gloves into which special soaps can be inserted is also effective. Used regularly every time you bathe, it will remove dirt and wastes, refine the pores and condition your skin. Rub it briskly across stubborn patches of cellulite on hips, thighs and upper arms .

You can also exercise in the bath to help tone up and firm muscles, especially in the legs and stomach. Just lie on your back and do alternate leg kicks 20 times as shown, or grip the sponge between your feet, raise your legs slowly and hold for a count of five, lower and repeat.

Hands and feet

While many of us pamper our faces, necks and bodies, we often overlook our hands and feet, which also need loving care. Perhaps because they are at the extremities of our limbs, we tend to take them for granted and they get neglected. But they are both essential for mobility and beauty. Dry uncared-for hands always reveal the tell-tale signs of age, and sore, aching feet, sometimes calloused or peppered with corns, will make you feel tired and old. For your overall health and fitness, it is important to look after them, so here's how:

Hands are exposed to the elements and pollutants every day: to the sun, heat, cold, wind, rain, alkaline soaps, household cleaners and detergents. You would never treat your face the way you abuse your poor hands. Yet they reflect your general level of health and even your character. Each hand, with its 27 bones, 26 muscles, blood vessels, nerves and skin, has different palm lines and finger prints and is a unique expression of you. The shape of your hand, the lines on your palm and how you use it are of interest to a palmist, and even to some psychologists. You use your hands for a whole range of movements and tasks, even for talking and communicating! Dry skin, callouses,

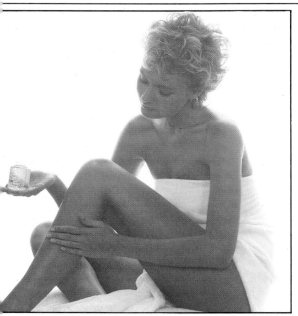

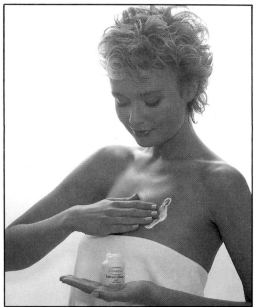

After a bath, gently rub a fragrant oil or cream into your skin to preserve its natural moisture and prevent it drying and flaking. This will keep skin looking younger.

ingrained dirt, age spots, cracked nails and uneven pigmentation not only make your hands look ugly but also make them look older. Here are the golden rules for looking after your hands to keep them in good condition with soft, youthful skin:

1 Wear rubber gloves for tasks involving water, such as washing clothes and dishes, and also for housework when using cleaners and chemicals.

2 Wear gloves for gardening to protect your hands from chemicals and earth.

3 Use a mild soap for washing your hands in warm, *not* hot, water.

4 Use a sunscreen to protect hands from sun-burn and brown liver spots — these are very ageing.

5 Wear warm gloves in cold weather.

6 Use a moisturising hand cream every day and after housework.

7 Treat your hands to a regular weekly manicure (see below).

Your nails also need care and attention to keep them healthy, strong and smooth. Most nail problems are caused by poor diet which is low in essential nutrients, but hormonal changes such as during pregnancy and among women taking the contraceptive pill can also affect the health of your nails. Only about half of each nail is visible — the rest extends below the skin down to the first joint. Your nail growth is affected by your age, the weather and how much you move your hands. About 5mm/¼in per month is normal, but nails will grow faster if you are young, the weather is warm and you exercise your fingers by typing or playing the piano regularly.

Protein, minerals (calcium, iron, iodine, sulphur and zinc) and vitamins A and B are all essential for healthy nails which are free from white spots, ridges and furrows. If your nails are fragile and split easily, you are probably deficient in vitamin A so include some cod liver oil, carrots, liver and yellow vegetables in your diet. If they are pale and brittle, you probably lack iron, so eat plenty of iron-rich foods, especially liver, apricots, eggs, molasses and brewers yeast. And if they are yellow and badly stained with nicotine, you should cut out smoking and your nails and hands will soon improve.

Home manicures are a good habit to adopt. You do not have to visit a beauty salon to obtain a good manicure. All you need are emery boards, nail remover polish, cotton wool pads, hand and cuticle creams, orange sticks and varnish. Set aside a quiet 30 minutes once a week for your hands and follow the simple steps outlined below:

Manicure routine

1 Remove any old nail polish with cotton wool soaked in varnish remover.

2 Using the smooth side of an emery board, carefully shape each nail. Always file from the sides towards the centre for a slender slightly oval shape, keeping the sides long to accentuate the length of your fingers. Keep all the nails a uniform length for neatness. They will look better than well-filed nails of different lengths.

3 Gently massage some cuticle cream or ordinary hand cream or oil around your cuticles and fingertips and then soak them in warm water for a few minutes. Pat dry.

4 Using an orange stick with a little cotton wool wound around the tip and moistened with warm soapy water or cuticle cream, carefully ease the cuticle of each nail gently back and scrape away any dead skin. Pat hands dry.

5 Massage your hands with moisturising hand cream or oil and then apply a coat of nail strengthener and varnish if wished. Or you can polish your nails with a buffer to make them glow.

Manicuring and caring for nails is an ancient art which has been practised by women for centuries all over the world. Even the ancient Egyptian queens were buried with their beautifully decorated manicure sets for use in the after-life. A weekly manicure will help keep your nails in good condition but it must be coupled with a healthy diet if they are to look smooth and pink as well as well-groomed. If your hands and nails are in bad shape you cannot expect instant results — it takes time for a new healthy nail to grow (nine months from its base) and for nails to reflect your change in diet and lifestyle. However, even the best-filed and well-cared-for nails can break on occasions and now you can buy special mending kits to repair them. A tiny dab of glue and varnish are usually enough to repair a broken or torn nail. Paint with a coat of coloured varnish and nobody will ever know the difference.

Feet that are well-maintained and in good condition are essential for effortless, graceful movement and good posture. Just 26 small bones, 33 joints, a series of arches, nerves, blood vessels and skin make up each foot and they can cause you a lot of unnecessary pain and discomfort if you fail to look after them, for these delicate bones support your body and powerful leg muscles. Foot problems are increasingly common and chiropodists estimate that about 90 per cent of these are caused by the wrong choice of footwear. Too many of us try to squeeze our feet into shoes that are too small, too pointed, too narrow or too high, with dire consequences for our feet. Callouses, corns, and blisters are the usual results, leading, in turn, to aching legs and back pain.

High heels are reponsible for a host of other problems, including shortening of the Achilles tendon, bad back posture and twisted ankles. In some cases, they may cause the pelvis to tilt in such a way that the muscles in the lower back area are affected and go into spasm. Fortunately, flatties are back in fashion, so high heels can be kept in the cupboard for more glamorous evening outings and special occasions. Your leg muscles are exercised more effectively in flat shoes as they go through a whole range of movements.

Choosing comfortable shoes can be quite a problem for most women, especially if they are fashion-conscious. Most shoes come in narrow fittings only, although the majority of women tend to have quite broad feet. Shop for shoes in the afternoon when your feet are warm and slightly swollen. The comfortable shoe you try on first thing in the morning may be agonising by the afternoon. Make sure that the shoe is at least 1cm/½in longer than your foot and that it fits comfortably with space on either side of the ball of the foot. Look for a heel height of 2·5 - 5cm/1 - 2in for comfort, good circulation and adequate exercising of leg muscles. Choose natural soft leather or suede in preference to synthetic materials which cause feet to swell and perspire. Never be tempted to buy a shoe with the idea of 'breaking it in'. If it is not comfortable when you try it on in the shop, it probably never will be — good shoes should feel right from the start.

Look after your feet by washing them daily in warm soapy water. Remove any hard, dead patches of skin by rubbing with a pumic stone. Pat dry and powder with talc or dusting powder. You can treat tired, aching feet to a tepid footbath of Epsom salts or a soothing commercial preparation. Alternatively, just add a few drops of lavender oil and allow feet to soak until they feel relaxed and revitalised. Always dry feet thoroughly afterwards to keep them free from infections. In warm weather wear open thong sandals to allow them to breathe more freely. They need plenty of air so walk around barefoot at home or wear cool, open shoes.

Beware of public swimming pools and changing rooms where you can pick up common infections such as athletes foot, verrucae and warts. You can buy special tinctures and powders for treating athletes foot and warts, but verrucae normally have to be removed professionally. Other foot problems include corns, bunions, callouses and chilblains. Badly-fitting shoes contribute to the formation of corns and bunions through excess pressure or friction. Although bunions have to be removed surgically, you can treat small corns yourself by rubbing gently with a pumice stone after soaking in warm water. A special corn pad will give relief, but if the condition worsens you should see a chiropodist and get it treated. Callouses can be controlled by regular washing and rubbing with a pumice stone. Rub in moisturising cream afterwards to soften the skin.

A weekly pedicure will also help keep feet in good condition. The principle is the same as for a manicure. Start by removing any old nail polish and then soak your feet in warm water for 10 minutes. Dip into cold water and then pat dry, especially between the toes. Now do the following:

Pedicure routine

1 Trim your nails evenly with scissors or nail-clippers. File them down smoothly with an emery board.

2 Gently massage some cuticle cream around the nails and ease back the cuticles with an orange stick, wrapped in cotton wool.

3 Treat patches of hard skin which the pumice has failed to remove with a special liquid remover.

4 Gently massage some moisturising cream into your feet and then polish your nails with varnish if wished.

Suncare

A glowing golden tan is considered both flattering and glamorous but too much sunshine can damage your skin and age it prematurely. If you want to avoid dry, wrinkled skin you should learn how to tan safely and painlessly without the discomfort and misery of red, burning skin and ugly blisters. For ultraviolet light is your skin's worst enemy, and it is probably more ageing then any other

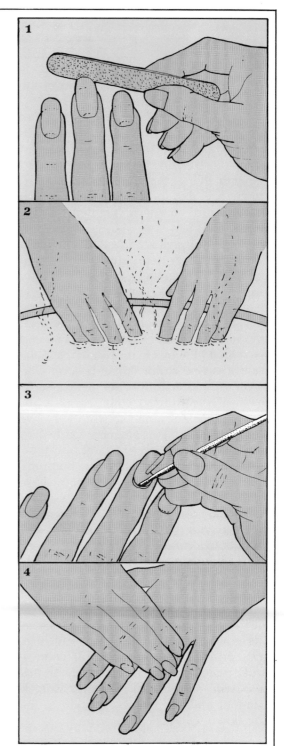

To manicure your nails yourself:
1 *File each nail with an emery board, working upwards from the sides into the centre to shape it prettily.*
2 *Immerse your fingers in warm water for a few minutes, and then pat dry.*
3 *Using an orange stick, tipped if wished with cotton wool and moistened with warm soapy water or cuticle cream, gently ease back each nail's cuticle and remove any pieces of dead skin.*
4 *Moisturise hands with hand cream to keep the skin really soft and smooth.*

single factor. To understand why this is so, you must examine the nature of the tanning process itself.

A tan is really your skin's way of protecting itself against the harmful effects of the sun. When you go outside on a hot sunny day a chain of events is precipitated beneath the surface of your skin. Deep down are the melanocyte cells which manufacture a dark pigment called melanin. When your skin is exposed to the sun's ultraviolet rays, the melanin travels upwards to the surface to prevent you burning, giving your skin a light brown colour. When the melanin is distributed evenly throughout your skin, you get a uniform overall tan, but when it is concentrated in certain areas, you end up with a blotchy tan or freckles as in the case of some very fair skinned people who never tan successfully. Your genetic background determines your capacity to produce melanin, and thus darker olive Mediterranean skins tan more easily than fairer Northern European ones.

Ultraviolet light is made up of tanning UV-A rays and burning UV-B rays. Most sunscreens block out the harmful UV-B rays while allowing the UV-A ones to tan you. A wide range of sunscreens and sunblocks is now available to protect your skin while you are out in the sun. The protective product you choose depends on your skin type and colouring. You will know from experience whether you tan easily or are inclined to burn and blister. By analysing your skin type accurately, you can decide how vulnerable you are and protect your skin accordingly. In this way you can choose the right suncare product and keep your exposure to the sun down to a realistic maximum.

Most sunscreens are graded according to a sun protection factor number on a scale descending from 15 to 2. The number you choose will be influenced by your colouring and past experiences of sun-bathing. Here is a rough guide:

1 If you are very pale with sensitive, delicate skin that is inclined to burn easily, possibly with a lot of freckles, then you may have to start with a strong sunblock, and then gradually work your way down through the sun protection numbers in the range of 15 to 8. Start with a high number and as your skin grows accustomed to the sun and your colour deepens, choose a lower number.

2 If you have normal skin that tans gradually but still needs some protection, then choose a factor number of 8, 7 or 6. This is only a moderate filter and you may have to use a higher factor number product on your face for added protection.

3 Good tanners who need only the minimum of protection can usually tan safely with a factor 4 product.

4 Lucky people with naturally dark olive skins that do not burn easily can get away with a factor number of 2 or 3. However, even their skin can get damaged or wrinkled eventually and they should be careful to protect their facial skin and moisturise after sun-bathing.

So you can see that the general rule is the hotter the sun and the more delicate your skin, the higher the sun protection factor number of the sunscreen you choose. Whatever your skin type, it is always advisable to start your tanning programme with a higher number and then gradually work down to a lower number which is right for your skin type. Remember to wear a sunscreen even when swimming as the ultraviolet rays can penetrate the water, and with the reflection off the sea or swimming pool you can get very burnt indeed, particularly on your shoulders and back. You can now buy special water-resistant sunscreens for this purpose.

To prevent uneven tanning, take care to apply the sunscreen uniformly, paying special attention to vulnerable areas such as breasts, nose, stomach, backs of knees, shoulders and feet. Make sure that your skin is fresh and clean when you do this, as most creams and lotions will not stick to oily sweaty skin and will afford little or no protection. If possible, choose a product that contains natural moisturisers such as cocoa butter, avocado, coconut oils and soothing aloe. Oil of bergamot is a common ingredient in many sun tan preparations but many women are allergic to this substance. If you are reaction-prone, then always check the ingredients on the bottle before you buy. Do not forget to protect your lips either as they do not produce melanin and can get very burnt and blistered. Use a special lipscreen in a handy swivel case and apply regularly.

You will also have to limit the amount

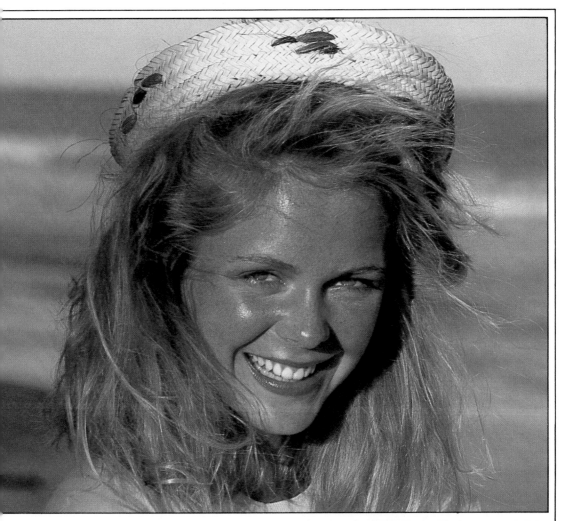

of time you spend in the sun — take it slowly and easily at first and gradually increase your exposure to sunlight by about 30 minutes each day. Start off by sunning yourself when the sun's ultraviolet rays are less intense, either before 11am or after 3pm. The middle of the day when the temperatures are hot and sunlight is very strong is the most dangerous period. Do not be fooled into staying out for longer on hazy days, or when the sun is shining brightly but a strong breeze makes you feel cool. The ultraviolet rays can still be sufficiently intense to give you nasty burns. Remember also that in tropical regions the sun's rays can penetrate even the shade to some extent, and that their intensity is doubled by any reflection off snow, water or even sand.

After-sun care, although it is neglected by many people, is just as important as suncare itself. You must apply moisturising creams and lotions to counteract the drying effects of the sun and keep your skin moist and supple. They will replace water loss and help you maintain your tan and keep

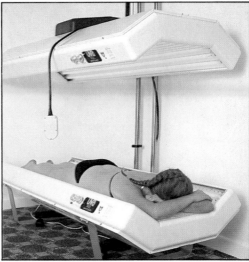

You can acquire a glowing golden tan outside in the sun or inside under a sun-lamp. Whichever way you choose to tan, make sure that you protect your skin with good sunscreen to prevent it burning and blistering. Do not overdo your tan as it can age your skin terribly, precipitating the formation of lines and wrinkles and cross-linking.

it longer. Take steps to prevent further drying by limiting the amount of soap you use when bathing as this can also deplete your skin of natural oils. Pat yourself dry with a towel and avoid rubbing yourself vigorously. To preserve the dark melanin pigment your skin has produced you must prevent it drying out, so apply a moisturising body cream or lotion regularly after bathing.

If you do get burnt, then use a soothing medicated after-sun preparation to take the heat and burning sensation out of your skin and make it less tender and sore. Gently rub in moisturising creams, or apply calamine lotion or a mixture of equal parts of baking soda (bicarbonate of soda) and water. Another natural and soothing preparation that sometimes brings relief is mashed cucumber pulp.

It must be pointed out that even if you tan easily and do not burn, there is still a risk of developing skin cancer, particularly if you live in a warm climate, such as Australia or some parts of the United States, and are exposed to a great deal of sun. Skin cancer is becoming more prevalent and thousands of new cases are treated every year. It sometimes occurs when new cells that have migrated upwards in the ultraviolet rays to the skin's surface do not die and are not shed by the skin in the normal way. Instead, they live on in the epidermis and the number of cells in this outer layer increases. If the skin is exposed to a lot more ultraviolet radiation these changed cells may eventually become a tumour. However, this may take several years, although it is sometimes less if you live in a very hot climate and are an ardent sun-worshipper. As the risks are always there, do take sensible precautions and always use a sunscreen to block out some of the harmful rays.

Hair care

Like an animal's fur coat, your hair reflects your general physical condition and health. When it is strong and glossy and full of body, then you are probably fit and healthy too, but if it is dull and lifeless then you might be below parr and not at your physical peak. Healthy hair should always look shiny and alive, whether it is long, short, curly, straight, thick or fine. However, the living part of the hair lies in the follicles beneath the surface of the skin, and the hair you see on your head is dead. A network of sebaceous glands and blood vessels supplies the growing hair with lubricating oil and nutrients which are essential for growth. The root of every hair is encased in a follicle, each with a tiny papilla at its base, which produces protein cells. Your hair consists of 97 per cent protein in the form of keratin, together with trace minerals and moisture.

Every strand of hair consists of three layers: the outer cuticle sheath, the inner cortex and the central medulla. The overlapping keratin cells of the cuticle protect the inner hair shaft. When magnified, they resemble fish scales which ideally should lie smoothly against each other so that your hair looks shiny and smooth. However, if they are raised or torn, perhaps because of bad brushing, harsh chemicals and dyes or over-heated rollers and excessive blow-drying, your hair will look dull and lifeless. So it is important to protect these cells that make your hair look glossy and healthy and reflect the light.

Most of us have between 90,000 and 150,000 hairs on our heads. Fine-haired blondes tend to have the most, with thicker haired brunettes coming next, and red-heads last. The colour of your hair is determined by the pigments in the cortex within each hair shaft — these may be black, red or yellow. Blonde hair has yellow pigment with traces of red; black and brown hair are both concentrations of black; and red hair comes from red pigment with traces of both yellow and black. When the cortex stops producing any pigment at all, the hair loses its natural colour and appears grey. Premature grey hairs can be triggered off by many factors — emotional shock and stress, mineral and vitamin deficiencies, particularly of vitamin B, a thyroid condition, or they may be simply hereditary.

Your hair grows at the rate of about 1.25cm/½in per month. It tends to grow faster during warm weather and when you are young. The quality of food you eat, the amount of exercise you take and your overall level of health and fitness can

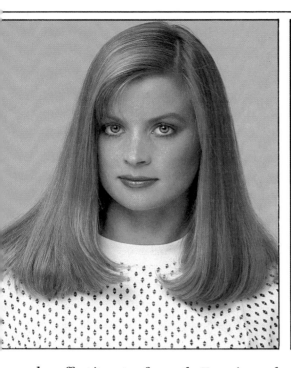

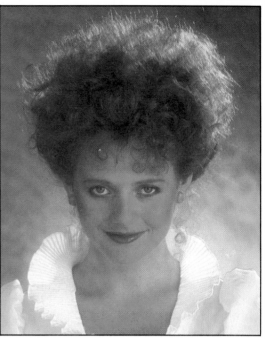

A good hair cut and effective conditioning will keep hair looking silky and soft. Whether your hair is straight or curly, it needs regular cutting and looking after to stay strong and healthy.

also affect its rate of growth. Exercise and massaging the scalp are both effective ways of stimulating circulation and ensuring a better supply of oxygen and nutrients to growing hair. And, contrary to what your hairdresser may have told you, cutting the hair will not increase its growth rate although it may keep the hair in better condition and free from split ends. For the hair grows from the follicle itself under your scalp as the papilla produces keratin and is nourished with nutrients and oxygen. The growth cycle is continuous and every day you shed between 100 and 200 hairs, but there is no need for anxiety as this is perfectly normal and new hairs are growing all the time to replace the ones you have lost. As you grow older or as your hair gets longer the rate of growth decelerates. The complete growth cycle for a single hair may last for anything between two and seven years, starting with the anagen phase when the hair follicle is expanding and oxygen and nutrients are utilised for growth, through the transitional catagen stage when the papilla stops producing keratin, to the final telogen stage when the follicle contracts and the hair is finally shed. Hair may be dislodged through shampooing and brushing, or as a result of physical and hormonal changes in the body, illness, shock or stress.

Type of hair

Your type of hair and whether it is curly, wavy, straight, thick or thin is part of the genetic make-up that you inherit. Its degree of curl is determined by the structure of the root and how it emerges from the follicle. If the root is smooth with the cells evenly distributed around the papilla, then your hair will be straight. However, if the root is distorted and the cell distribution is uneven, then the hair will kink and bend as it grows out of the follicle and your hair will be curly or wavy.

Normal hair is neither too dry nor too greasy and will last from five to eight days without washing. It is usually easy to look after with plenty of healthy shine and bounce.

Dry hair, which often lacks lustre and is very fine and flyaway, is prone to split ends and needs careful conditioning. A good balsam or protein shampoo and conditioner can help coat the hair shafts to give them strength and align the scales on the cuticles. If your hair falls into this category, you must take care when blow-drying it and avoid harmful chemical treatments which might do further damage.

Greasy hair is caused by over-active sebaceous glands which stimulate and release too much oil. Just one or two days after washing, it can appear lank and lifeless. A good diet, which is low in fats, sugars and refined foods, and regular washing with a mild shampoo will help improve its condition. Lemon shampoos and conditioners are especially effective in treating it as they cut down oil *and* leave the hair shiny and manageable.

Fine hair tends to be more common among blondes than brunettes. Soft and delicate, it needs regular shampooing and careful conditioning to give it adequate protection from the effects of the sun, enthusiastic brushing and blow-drying. A good cut will help add fullness and body. Because it is so thin and fine it is often difficult to set and to keep in a certain style.

Straight hair is usually thick and tough and easy to manage. It usually contains dark pigment, especially if it is very thick and strong. Regular shampooing and conditioning will give it gloss and bounce and a good cut will make it hang well. Many people, of course, get bored with straight hair and opt for a perm to give it more body and curl. It is strong enough to cope with this form of treatment.

Curly hair needs regular conditioning to keep it soft and shiny and to prevent any wiriness. A good hairdresser will follow the line of the curl or layer it for stunning results. Mild shampoos and regular cutting will prevent it becoming wild and frizzy.

Washing

Beautiful, well-conditioned hair must be kept clean, and while some people find that they can get by on just one shampoo a week, others wash their hair every day. It depends on your type of hair — whether it is naturally dry or greasy, its cut, general condition and the environment to which it is subjected. If you live in a city your hair will probably need more frequent washing than country hair, as it is bombarded daily by dirt and traffic fumes. The best guide is to wash hair whenever it starts to look and feel dirty, greasy, dull or unkempt, which may take anything from one to seven days. Clean, soft hair with natural shine and body will feel right and give you more confidence than dirty hair.

Choosing the right shampoo is always a matter of trial and error. There is such a wide choice of creams, lotions, gels and pastes, ranging from mild natural ones to harsher detergent-based products, that it can be baffling. Most of these are fortified with all sorts of different ingredients, including herbs, fruits, balsam, protein, vegetable oils, egg, lemon, beer and flowers. The best guide is to analyse your hair type and to buy a shampoo that is formulated specially to enhance and condition your sort of hair. Thus there are preparations for treating dry and greasy hair, tinted, coloured, lightened, bleached and straightened hair. By shopping around and trying different products you will soon discover what suits you best. Many hairdressers think that it is a good idea not to stick to just one shampoo but to alternate two or three different ones. Your hair can change according to your diet, your level of exercise, the season, your emotions and the weather. The shampoo that is right for your hair when it is cold in winter or when you are working hard, under stress and eating filling, warming foods, may not be right in the summer months when you are more relaxed, eating plenty of fresh vegetables and fruit, and are exercising regularly. When you go away on holiday to a warmer climate and spend more time in the sun and the water, you will probably need another shampoo to protect your hair from the drying effects of the sea and sun.

Many shampoos contain conditioners as well as cleansing agents in order to make hair softer, more shiny and manageable. Always opt for a mild shampoo, preferably pH balanced, that will protect your hair's natural acidity. Harsh chemical shampoos can strip away this acid mantle and make hair appear dull and lifeless. Herbal shampoos enliven and condition hair; balsam adds thickness and body by coating the hair shafts and making them stronger; lemon combats oiliness and leaves hair fresh, shining and smelling fragrant; camomile lightens hair and is suitable for blondes; and protein and egg-based shampoos thicken and protect dry, damaged hair. They may be absorbed by the hair shafts and help smooth the cuticles' covering scales to make hair look shinier and softer.

You can experiment with making your own shampoos. Mix an infusion of

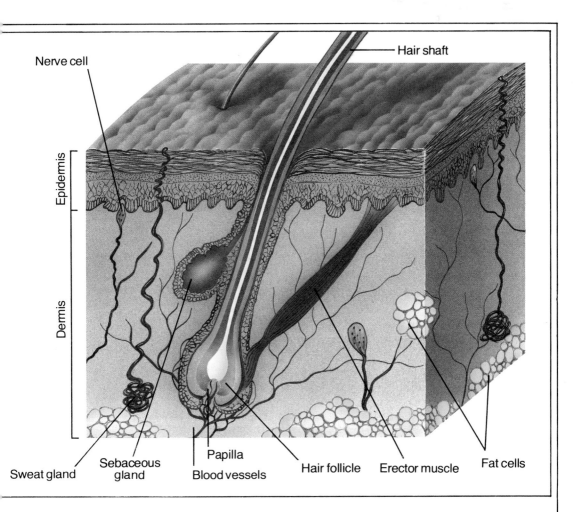

Nerve cell

Epidermis

Dermis

Hair shaft

Sweat gland

Sebaceous gland

Papilla

Blood vessels

Hair follicle

Erector muscle

Fat cells

stimulating herbs, such as rosemary, thyme or white nettle with some pure soap shampoo and massage well into the scalp. Or add beaten egg yolks or an infusion of camomile flowers. When shampooing, always massage the scalp thoroughly to remove dead cells and stimulate circulation. Then rinse well to remove any traces of shampoo and leave hair feeling really clean and the scalp slightly squeaky when you rub it. If you don't wash the shampoo out completely it will make your hair dull or greasy. You can add a little vinegar or lemon juice to the final rinse to add lustre and shine.

Conditioning

A good conditioner will coat the hair shafts and protect them from damage. It will make your hair feel softer and silkier and reduce static electricity between the hair and the comb, making it easier to get rid of tangles. Each hair is coated with a fine film, usually of protein or balsam, which smoothes down the cuticle, protecting it from moisture loss and adding strength and thickness. Conditioners come in many forms — as instant cream rinses whose

This cross-section through the scalp shows the structure of a single hair shaft and the surrounding skin. It is fed with nutrients such as protein by the blood vessels and oil by the sebaceous gland.

fast action means that you simply rub them into your hair after rinsing, leave for two to five minutes and then wash off; or as special protein packs and deep treatment oil and wax conditioners which take about 20 minutes to act. These special treatments are ideal for damaged, tinted and permed hair, making it more resilient, glossy and manageable. However, they should be used only once every two or three weeks and not every time you wash your hair. Use a cream rinse in between treatments.

Setting and drying

The best and safest way to dry hair is to leave it to dry naturally without any artificial heat which can be damaging. But sophisticated hair cuts which often need coaxing into a particular style, and a busy modern lifestyle usually dictate the use of heated rollers and dryers. Blow-drying is probably the most popular method as it is quick and easy and gives a natural look, giving hair bounce and lift. Never allow the dryer to become over-heated — always use warm, not hot, air or it will damage your hair and cause the ends to become dry, brittle and split. Wait for the hair to dry a little before you start — wrap it up in a towel for about five minutes to speed up the process. Use a brush to curl and style the hair and hold the dryer at least 15cm/6in away from your head as you work, moving the dryer around all the time so that the heat is not concentrated on too small an area for too long. The result should last for two to three days before it starts to drop out of shape.

Rollers are another way of setting hair, of course, and may be the traditional sort or special heated ones. Heated rollers are useful for styling hair that is over one-day old since washed and needs coaxing back into shape. Always protect the hair by wrapping some tissue paper round it as the hot rollers will dry out and damage the hair if used directly on it. For tight curls, wrap only a little hair tightly around each roller, whereas for looser more natural waves, wind more hair loosely around the rollers. Allow heated rollers to cool before removing them and brushing out the hair.

Many women advocate the use of curling tongs for styling hair, especially for fringes and small curls to frame the face, but these are more damaging than either dryers or rollers as they can scorch your hair. If you insist on using them, choose teflon or plastic coated ones to minimise the damage and use for a few seconds only or your hair will frizzle.

Special hair treatments

Most of us get bored with the colour or appearance of our hair at some time or another and long to change it. It is amazing how refreshing a new hair style can be and the difference it makes to our self-image. Nowadays we can change our hair in so many ways — by colouring, tinting or streaking it; by curling, waving or straightening it; or simply by cutting and styling it. However, many of these treatments are potentially damaging to

hair and necessitate some extra-careful shampooing, conditioning, drying and brushing afterwards to compensate for them. Here is a survey of some of the most common treatments available.

Permanent waves are softer and less damaging than ever before, and harsh chemicals are being used less. Although there are many home perms available, it is safer to go to a hairdresser and have it done by a professional, especially as not everybody's hair can take a perm successfully and you may end up with an unmanageable frizz. Basically, the thicker and coarser your hair and the more healthy it is, the better its chances of taking a perm well and holding it longer. The cut and the shape should be right also and you will have to ask your hairdresser whether you should think about changing your style if you want a perm. If possible, always opt for one of the new soft perms which are gentler and more flattering. They are not so damaging to your hair's natural pH balance, and with regular cutting your hair should stay in good condition with few split ends. When hair is permed the chemical bonds within the protein molecules are broken and remade to change the shape and pattern of the hair shafts, so some damage is inevitable although many modern perms contain special conditioning agents to combat this.

Straightening is really the perming process done in reverse, although it is much more complex and should only be attempted by professionals and never at home. Unlike perming, which can be practised two or three times a year, straightening is a once-a-year-only pro-cedure. Special chemicals are used, usually ammonium or sodium bisulfate, or sodium hydroxide. You will need to protect your hair afterwards from the harmful effects of sun and sea-water.

Colouring hair is the easiest way of changing its appearance, especially if you use a temporary rinse which lasts for one shampoo only but gives subtle highlights and rich, deep tones. Gone are the days of peroxide blondes and blue rinses — today's colours are more natural and subtle with the emphasis on natural vegetable dyes, especially henna and camomile. The secret is never to fight your natural colouring — you can usually lighten your hair by two to three shades without it looking odd, but you should never attempt to go darker, or indeed to go completely blonde if you have naturally dark hair and skin colouring. The results can be very bizarre. Rather than attempting to completely change your natural colouring, aim to enhance and improve on it, or to boost lacklustre and greying hair. Experiment with a temporary colour rinse before you go the whole way and use a permanent colourant — you may not like the result! The best shades to choose are honey, hazel, chestnut and russet to add gleaming highlights and a wonderful glow to your hair.

These temporary rinses have to be renewed when you rewash your hair, most lasting for one shampoo only. They work by coating the outside of the cuticle with colour without penetrating the hair shaft itself. They often contain some softening conditioners and are non-damaging, and although they cannot cover grey hairs they do help to disguise them.

Like temporary colour rinses, semi-permanent colourings do not contain peroxide and can be applied at home. Although they are more intense, their effects last only through four or five shampoos before fading. They penetrate the hair shaft slightly but the overall effect is usually gentle, lightening or enhancing your natural colour within a range of given colour tones. Many are conditioning and will leave your hair feeling silky and glossy.

Permanent colourings should always be applied by a professional as they penetrate the hair shaft, stripping away its natural colour and altering its structure. Metallic and analine dyes and bleaches are usually used and these can be damaging to hair, making it dry and brittle. Careful conditioning is needed to keep this sort of coloured hair manageable and smooth. Another disadvantage is that as the hair grows, the roots will need retouching as your natural colour begins to show. Vegetable dyes are the best way to colour hair permanently as they are non-toxic and do not contain chemicals. Many, such as henna, have been used safely for thousands of years without fear of allergy. Henna powder can make fair hair a glorious Titian or give dark hair a deep chestnut, reddish glow. Always try it out on a few strands of hair before applying overall as it can turn some mousy and light hair an unattractive shade of orange. Once applied, it will last several months before it needs retouching. It also acts as an excellent conditioner for hair but should be applied by a top colourist to achieve the right intensity and tone.

Camomile is another natural herbal colouring and is used to lighten fair or blonde hair. The result is always natural with subtle streaks and highlights. Usually several applications are necessary to achieve the required colour and effect. You can go to a colourist or try making an infusion of dried camomile flowers (about 30ml/2 tablespoons flowers to 550ml/1 pint boiling water) and simmering for 15 minutes. Strain and cool and use as a final rinse after shampooing your hair.

Streaking (top) and colouring (below) are both ways of enlivening your hair and giving it a new look. For permanent colours, both should be done by a professional in a salon and not attempted yourself at home.

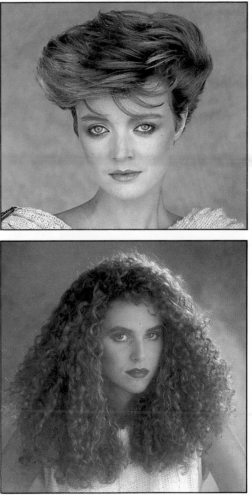

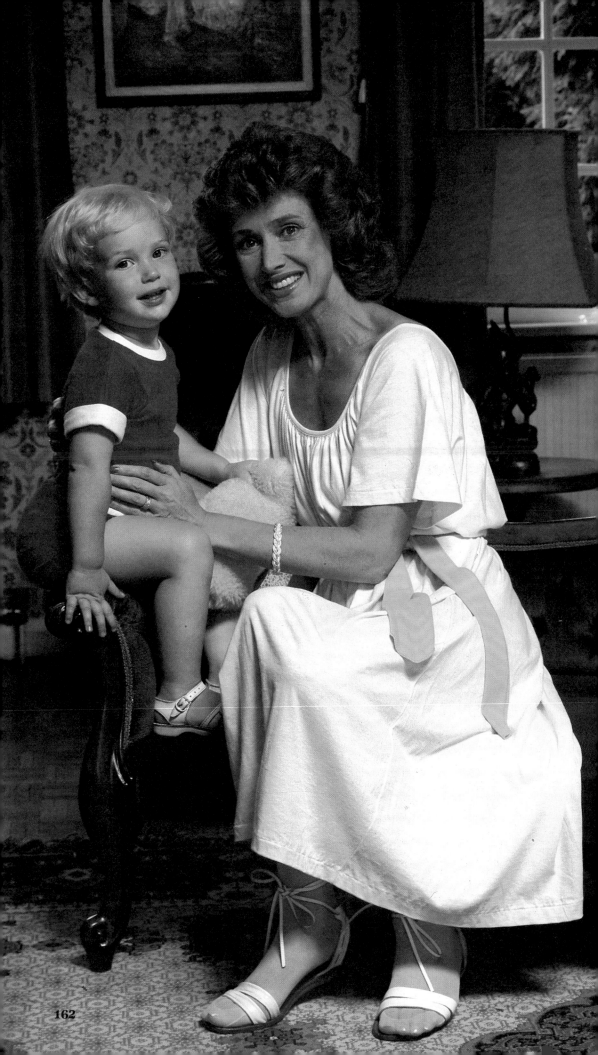

Jan Leeming

Jan Leeming combines a successful career as a newsreader on British television with running a home and bringing up her young son. She lives with her husband Patrick and two-year-old Jonathan in a quiet Buckinghamshire village, and most days she commutes into London for work. Fit and slim, she seems to thrive on an incredibly busy timetable, which most women would find daunting.

"I lead a very ordinary life. I don't have a lot of time to spend on myself because I am so busy. I feel younger and have more energy now than I did 10 years ago. Life is very exciting at the moment, especially with Jonathan. Although I probably need to relax more, I haven't got time. I think I've watched television about twice in the last eighteen months! My relaxation is my son. When I get a day off, we just play together and enjoy ourselves."

Jan does all the shopping and cooking herself and is a firm believer in eating a healthy diet with plenty of natural wholefoods. "I always buy whole grain bread and whole grain spaghetti, brown sugar etc. Everybody really has to educate themselves to healthy eating. I don't eat a special diet but I used to be fat and have got accustomed to watching my weight and the sort of foods I eat. Once you get to your ideal weight it is easy to stay there if you eat healthy foods. A homeopath told me that you need a raw salad every day, and I always eat one with plenty of fresh green pepper, shredded raw carrot and a selection of vegetables. I like fish but I don't eat much meat. I've cut down gradually over the years and never eat veal or lamb. People argue that it is expensive to eat well — it's actually cheaper than buying convenience foods. It worries me that a lot of trace elements and minerals are disappearing from our food, and so I grow my own fresh herbs as they are a wonderful source of vitamins and minerals."

When Jan became pregnant she followed a healthy eating plan and exercised regularly. "I didn't touch any spirits at all, although I did enjoy the occasional glass of white wine. I still do all the exercises for my stomach. They helped me to regain my figure after Jonathan was born. I hate diets and I love good food, but if I eat a lot, I make up for it the next day by eating very plain, healthy food.

"I was very happy during my pregnancy. I ate well and laughed a lot. I'm glad that I had a child in my late thirties as I doubt that having children in my twenties would have been good for them or for me. I am now better equipped to cope with motherhood and can enjoy it more. I'm very lucky that I have a good career, and Jonathan is a wonderful *addition* to my life."

Jan takes vitamins every day to supplement her diet. "I take vitamins B,C,E and ginseng. I think that they help to keep me healthy and give me more energy." She believes in natural medicine and homeopathy and tries very hard not to take drugs unless they are absolutely essential.

Her beauty routine is simplicity itself, as she explains in her new book *Jan Leeming's Practical Book of Beauty* published by Weidenfeld. "I use products containing plant extracts on my skin, and it takes me 10 minutes to put my make-up on in the morning, and five minutes to take it off and put my creams on at night." Jan thinks that good skincare is important for every woman and will help keep you looking younger. Her other tip for staying youthful is to: "Eat healthy food, get enough sleeep and look after your body. Then you can stave off the years."

163

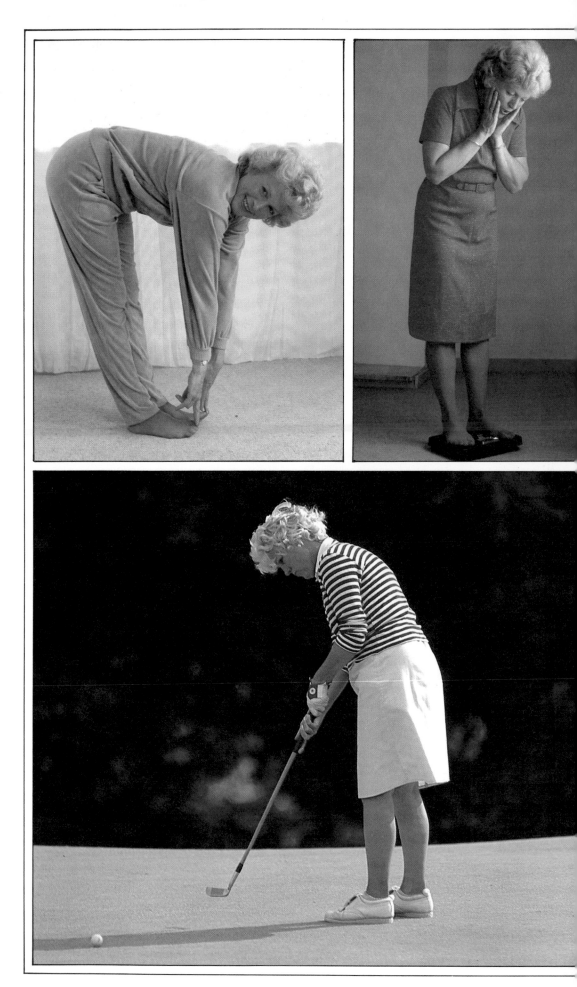

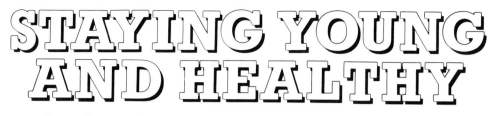

STAYING YOUNG AND HEALTHY

You need to take good care of your body and stay in shape if you want to be healthy and slow down the inevitable ageing process in your body. So learn how to look after yourself in order to stay young in body and mind.

Staying healthy

Good health is any woman's greatest asset and well worth taking good care of. Health care is becoming increasingly important as 50 per cent of deaths in the Western world are now attributable to 'lifestyle' diseases. The food you eat, the exercise you take, the job you have and the amount of stress to which you are subjected all affect your general health and life expectancy. Heart disease, lung cancer and strokes, once thought of as the exclusive preserve of men, are becoming increasingly common in women too as they lead more responsible and stressful lives. Most modern women run a family *and* a job and they have little time for relaxation. They are often too busy taking care of others to make time for themselves. But you alone have to take responsibility for your health by improving the quality of your life and by practising some preventive medicine. It is better to take postive steps to stay fit and healthy and to have regular medical check-ups to confirm this than to wait until you are ill before you go to the doctor.

A self-help approach to your health can literally work wonders when it comes to preventing disease or identifying it in its early stages before it is too late to treat it effectively. If you have followed the general guidelines set out in the previous chapters and have developed new eating and exercise habits, then you are already on the road to good health. A poor lifestyle proffers the geatest risks of all. Improving your diet, increasing your activity and exercise levels, eliminating tension and stress, relaxing more and changing your smoking and drinking habits are all beneficial and you will feel healthier and more energetic.

But we usually tend to notice our health only when we feel ill, and take it for granted when we are well. As you can see, staying healthy depends on far more than just not having a headache or a cold or a virus; on the contrary, it is being fit, in good shape with glowing skin, glossy hair, sleeping well and feeling emotionally content, if not high. You cannot be fit and healthy if you are depressed, tense or irritable. Most people find that the slimmer and healthier they become, the more they enjoy their lives as they feel better inside and have a higher self-image. Often they discover that they can achieve more, and are more successful and self-confident as their body-image improves.

Looking after your body is not vain or narcissistic — it makes good sense. It is a positive and valuable approach to your own mental and physical health and also a voyage of self-discovery as you learn more about your body and thereby about yourself. We have tended to ignore our health in the past, but now thousands of women are becoming aware of the benefits of being strong, fit and healthy and are experiencing a new lease of life. Exercise, fitness and good diet have added an exciting new dimension to their lives. So it is worth taking the time and trouble to stay healthy and prevent your body going wrong. If you maintain it well and service it regularly it will stay in first class condition and you will feel and look better and healthier as a result. Being aware of your body and your emotional state of mind enables you to detect when something goes wrong and to recognise the danger-signs and act positively to restore good health.

Regular self-examination and body maintenance are the corner-stones of preventive medicine as more women are coming to realise. Most of us now examine our breasts for possible lumps and have regular cervical smear tests as a matter of course, and with breast and cervical cancer being among the leading causes of death in middle-aged women, this is highly desirable. But good health also depends on keeping teeth and gums

165

healthy, staying slim and supple, and having a regular menstrual cycle. Look at our table of health and fitness to assess your own health. Don't cheat — answer the questions honestly and decide how healthy and fit you really are. Then look at our short guide to the warning signs of ill-health.

1 Do you feel supple and mobile without any stiffness in any limbs or joints?
2 Do you ever feel anaemic, listless or lacking in energy?
3 Do you have trouble getting to sleep, or wake frequently throughout the night?
4 Are you often constipated?
5 Do you ever suffer from indigestion or stomach aches?
6 Do you often experience headaches or migraine?
7 Are your periods regular?
8 Do you ever suffer from premenstrual tension or water retention?
9 Do you sometimes feel depressed, low and lacking in vitality?
10 Do you smoke, drink or take any drugs (tranquillisers, amphetamines etc?)
11 Do you feel that you look good with a slim body, healthy skin and hair?
12 Do you suffer from back ache?
13 Do you feel breathless when you run, walk or cycle even a short distance?
14 Do you examine your breasts for any lumps regularly?
15 Do you use dental floss to attack plaque?

Teeth and gums

Healthy teeth and gums are rare among older women, and even young women and children now suffer from tooth decay and gum disease if they consume too many sugary, over-refined foods. Our Western diet and generally poor dental hygiene mean that we do not take enough care of our teeth, yet nobody wants to wear dentures or lose their teeth. You may be surprised to learn that most dental problems are due to unhealthy gums — not bad teeth. Teeth are made of the hardest substance in your body, calcium phosphate, and they are naturally strong. They were not designed, however, for a diet that is high in refined sugar and white flour. Harmful bacteria are attracted to the food residue left in your mouth after eating these foods and they gradually attack your teeth, leading eventually to gum disease and tooth decay. Regular brushing and dental flossing help control plaque and reduce the risk of decay. Unfortunately, brushing alone is not very effective as a disclosing tablet will reveal. It looks a little horrific but the areas of plaque and food residue that remain after brushing will look purple or red. Brushing each tooth individually in the direction in which it grows with a good toothbrush will cut down on plaque but flossing backwards and forwards between the teeth is also essential. Use the unwaxed floss once every day and make it a regular habit.

Good posture

The word 'posture' has an old-fashioned ring about it but it is vital for good health. Bad posture can lead to fatigue, back ache, foot problems, poor breathing and digestion, and even arthritis in later life. Slouching forwards with hunched shoulders does not do a lot for your looks either, and you will find that you look taller and slimmer when you stand up straight with stomach tucked in and shoulders straight and down. Your spine was designed to have an easy alignment, your back muscles supporting the spinal column and preventing the nerves from becoming trapped.

If you do not carry your spine correctly, the vertebrae will get compressed, causing friction and tension and maybe even bone or joint displacement. But because most people have bad posture they often feel uncomfortable when they throw their shoulders back, press their lower back inwards and lift their chest. It does not take long to get into the habit if you are aware of posture and practise it regularly. It will soon come naturally to you. You will find that you carry yourself more gracefully as a result, that you will breathe more deeply and fully as your lungs work more efficiently, and you are less likely to experience back pain or aching feet.

Wearing high heels contributes to bad posture as they throw your weight artificially forwards, shifting your centre of gravity and throwing your spine into an artificial curve. Because your weight is not evenly distributed across the base of each foot, you may develop callouses and curled-up toes. Wearing flatter and low-heeled shoes helps enormously, and stretching exercises will ease out your spine and develop stronger muscles and better posture.

Anaemia

Feeling tired or listless, lacking in energy? If you suspect that you are anaemic you should ask your doctor for a blood test. Anaemia is a condition which affects your body when it is deficient in red blood cells and thus does not get its full quota of nutrients and oxygen to perform all its functions efficiently. Most low haemoglobin counts are due to lack of iron, although they may also be caused by vitamin deficiency. A heavy loss of blood, especially during a period, may sometimes lead to anaemia, and you will have to take iron supplements or eat iron-rich foods, such as liver and green vegetables. Vitamin C in the form of citrus fruits is essential too as it helps your body to absorb iron. Vitamin B12 (cyanocobalamin) is also useful as it plays an important role in the production of red blood cells and is often known as the anti-anaemia vitamin. Fatigue, depression and insomnia are related to its deficiency in the body.

Health hazards

Social habits such as smoking and alcohol both constitute major health hazards as they undermine your health gradually and may even lead to serious illness and death, either directly or indirectly as they are contributory factors in many modern killer diseases. Although they may start as a harmless social thing to do, both can become addictive, and a drinking problem can wreck your life, ruining your health, your family and other relationships and your career. The other major health hazard discussed here is drugs—not hard drugs like cocaine and heroin (although these of course are highly dangerous) but the seemingly innocuous pills you may take regularly to send you to sleep or pep you up or calm you down. Thousands of women are now dependent on these drugs for their mental well-being but they are probably doing them more harm than good and solve nothing in the long-term. So read on and discover whether your indulgence in any one of these habits is harming your health.

Smoking is a causative factor in chronic bronchitis, heart disease and lung cancer, and all these conditions are becoming more frequent among women as well as men, as more women smoke. There is no doubt whatsoever that if you smoke your chances of getting one of these serious diseases is greatly increased, and the more you smoke the greater the risks become. And even if you manage to avoid these health problems, you may still contract cancer of the mouth, throat, oesophagus, pancreas or bladder. If you smoke while you take the contraceptive pill, your chances of having a heart attack are increased 12 fold over those of a woman who neither smokes nor takes the Pill.

Cigarettes contain three active ingredients: nicotine, tar and carbon-monoxide. When you light up a cigarette and inhale the smoke, it is taken down into your lungs and the nicotine acts as a stimulant to the tiny receptors in your respiratory tract. It also affects your brain, making you more alert and receptive with greater powers of concentration. Thus many people tend to reach for a cigarette while they are working hard to focus their minds on the problem in hand. They find that they can sustain mental activity for longer periods if they smoke a cigarette. However, on the debit side, nicotine also narrows the coronary arteries leading to the heart which supply it with essential nutrients and oxygen, and it raises your blood pressure and the cholesterol levels in your body by causing a hormone to be released into your blood stream, thus increasing the risk of heart disease.

The tar damages the cilia (fine hairs) that line your windpipe and bronchial passages, leading to a build-up of particles, debris and mucus which cannot be removed in the normal way by coughing. Eventually your whole respiratory system becomes damaged, blocked and infected and this may lead to chronic bronchitis, emphysema or lung cancer.

Thus the psychological benefits you may feel you receive from smoking are far outweighed by the damage it can do to your health. Every cigarette you light is potentially damaging to your body. There is no point eating healthy foods, exercising regularly and generally striving to get fit and lead a more healthy lifestyle if you continue to smoke. Smoking can affect the way you look outside as well as how you function inside. Because the benzopyrene in cigarettes depletes your body's supply of vitamin C, which is necessary for sustaining

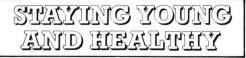

healthy collagen in your skin, smoking can damage and age your skin, leading to cross-linking and premature wrinkling.

Alcohol can be enjoyable in moderation but you should always remember that it is potentially addictive and damaging to your health. Because it affects your nervous system, heavy drinkers and alcoholics may eventually experience brain damage, poor coordination and loss of memory. Heart disease is another hazard as heavy drinking may lead to a rise in blood levels of triglycerides (the fatty substances that help promote heart disease) and even damage to the heart muscles themselves. Even moderate drinkers run a greater risk than non- drinkers of suffering a stroke. The other killer disease associated with high levels of drinking is cirrhosis of the liver — the death rate from this has been rising steadily over the last 20 years.

It was once thought unladylike and unfeminine for women to drink but now that they are working in more responsible, stressful jobs and society's norms have changed, more and more women are drinking socially. In fact, one quarter of the alcoholics in the West are now women, most of them under 40 years old. They tend to become problem drinkers either through stress and excessive pressures at work or at home, or through boredom. Many women who stay at home and feel frustrated that they do not have a career or a rewarding life, turn to drink as a means of escape. Feeling isolated and depressed may easily cause a moderate drinker to become a heavy drinker and to reach for the bottle as soon as she feels down and needs a pick-me-up. But when you find that you cannot get through the day without a few drinks to help you along, your skin starts to look puffy and blotchy, your eyes blood-shot and little broken veins appear on your face, you really should ask yourself whether you are growing dependent on alcohol and using it as a crutch.

What most people don't seem to realise is that alcohol is potentially dangerous and addictive. The more you drink and the more accustomed you become to it, the less you will feel its effects and you will have to drink larger amounts to receive the required

'high' or release from your problems and worries. Your level of drinking may seem perfectly acceptable and normal to you although it might appear excessive to an ordinary drinker. Reaching automatically for a drink when you are tired, under stress, upset, worried or bored can lead to a serious drinking problem, especially as a woman's tolerance of alcohol in her body is not so high as that of a man. Even though you may drink exactly the same quantity of alcohol as a man, you will become intoxicated more quickly as your body contains less water. This means that the alcohol in your system is in a more concentrated form and it takes less time for damage to vital organs to occur. Liver damage in heavy women drinkers takes less time and fewer drinks than in men. If you start to eat less, alienate yourself from family and friends and drink secretly, then you should seek professional help or guidance.

Accepting some responsibility for your health and respecting your body involves cutting down on your alcohol intake, even if you are only a light or moderate drinker. You will feel so much better as a result — you will be lighter-headed, more alert, you will think more clearly, your skin will also be clearer and glowing and your eyes will not look sore, tired or bloodshot.

Drugs, their use and abuse, are now more widespread than ever before. There seem to be drugs to cure almost any pain, sickness or psychological problem, and many are readily available over the counter in drugstores and chemists as well as on prescription from your doctor. More women are becoming pill-poppers — they need drugs to calm them down, pep them up, send them to sleep, relax them and cure minor aches and pains. Many are now on long-term medication so that eventually they become addicted to barbiturates, amphetamines or tranquillisers to such an extent that they feel they cannot face life without them. Although it may be beneficial to take sleeping pills or tranquillisers over a short period of a week or two to form new better sleeping habits or as a temporary measure to help you over an emotional crisis, it should not be prolonged over many weeks or months, as psychologically you may grow to depend on them for your mental and emotional well-being.

More women are at risk than men, as they take more of these drugs, especially tranquillisers, which are particularly debilitating and habit-forming. Although they may seem to make you feel calmer and more in control of your life, they cannot attack or solve the causes of your stress, worries or anxieties — they only treat the symptoms. And while you take them, you are not really in control at all as you may lose the power of objective decision-making and clear thinking. If you want to lead a more healthy lifestyle using more natural methods to cope with stress, such as relaxation and exercise, you must see that it is not safe to use artificial chemical means over a long period of time to alter your state of mind.

Alternative medicine

Although orthodox medicine is making great advances in the treatment of many diseases more and more people are turning to practitioners in alternative medicine, either to help prevent illness or to treat minor ailments. The attraction of alternative medicine lies in its more personal, positive approach for it takes you as a person, into account, as well as your symptoms. Whereas a medical doctor would be concerned to treat the isolated pain and symptoms of your problem, an alternative medicine practitioner would delve deeper into the causes to discover why and how you became ill, and then would try to restore your whole body to health. More natural methods than surgery and drugs are emphasised, especially manipulation of bones and joints, herbal remedies, a healthy diet and lifestyle, and the use of essential aromatic oils.

If you are interested in treating your body in a more natural, gentle way and dislike taking powerful drugs, often with unpleasant side-effects, you might like to try this branch of medicine which exists on the fringe of orthodox practice. Many doctors no longer scoff at such forms of treatment as acupuncture, osteopathy, chiropractic and homeopathy and recognise that they may complement the work they do themselves. Thus they are fast becoming an increasingly respectable form of health care with an important role to play in preventive medicine and drugless therapy. Always make sure that the practitioner you consult is properly qualified and belongs to one of the professional bodies or assocations. In this way, you can be assured that he has a minimum standard of training and knowledge in his chosen field.

Followers and practitioners of alternative medicine believe in the health-giving life-force of every body which encourages the body to fight disease and endows it with a form of energy for this purpose. Any disease or sickness is viewed as a disturbance of this basic force and may spring from imbalances within the body itself. If these are corrected, the life-force can be encouraged to restore it to health and wholeness. Alternative medicine stresses health, not illness, and attempts to maintain good health so that breakdowns and imbalances do not occur and visits to the doctor are unnecessary.

You are encouraged to get to know and understand your body, its physical and emotional patterns, so that you are aware when something goes wrong and can take steps to prevent it happening. By leading a healthy lifestyle, eating a nutritious diet, relaxing and exercising and treating your body naturally, you are better equipped to stay healthy and vital.

Many people are a little sceptical about alternative medicine and its methods but if it gives positive results, relieves your pain or discomfort and makes you feel better, then you should not dismiss it lightly. Use it to complement the treatment and attention that you receive from your doctor. It can work with, and not against, the traditional methods of medicine.

Staying young

If we could retain the glowing skin and physical vitality of youth and at the same time enjoy the benefits of our years of experience we would have, in middle age, an ideal situtation. But inexorably our bodies age with the years and there is no mysterious fountain of youth.

At the present time there is so much emphasis on youth that the ageing crisis starts earlier — in our late twenties and early thirties — and lasts longer. And the belief that young is beautiful, old is ugly is reinforced in much of what we read, see and hear through the media. We need to question this for there are real, tangible advantages in growing old, as well as disadvantages. Most women in their thir-

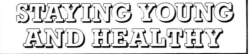
ties will admit that their late teens and early twenties those years of visible youth, were not years of unadulterated bliss.

This does not mean that we should resign ourselves to ageing for there are a great many things we can do to slow down the ageing process, just as physical neglect of our bodies and lack of mental stimulation will hasten the onset of old age. The aim of many of the 'youth preserving' procedures mentioned here is not so much to prolong life as to make it more vital and rewarding. As one gerontologist has said, 'There is every indication that if we arrive at old age skipping rather than crawling we can modify the effects of ageing.'

Most of the body's organs age and deteriorate without us being particularly aware of the process. We may not have the physical stamina we had at, say 18, but usually we accept this as part and parcel of 'maturity'. There is one feature, however, which can — and often does — show our age in an obvious way, and that is our skin; for although the skin's ageing process is really no different from anywhere else in the body, it can be much faster. Just how fast depends on a number of factors of which probably the most important is our genetic inheritance. If your mother and grandmothers had youthful, glowing skin at the age of 60, chances are that, with reasonable skin care, you will too, and vice versa.

How the skin ages

Pinch a patch of skin on your hand and after a second or two release it. The skin of a teenager will rapidly return to its original shape, but older skin will take several seconds longer. This is because as skin ages it loses it elasticity and becomes wrinkled and crêpey. And this is not all. As we grow older, cell growth slows down causing, among other things, a build-up of dead cells on the surface which discolourations begin to develop into the blotchy freckle-like patches called liver spots. Hormonal levels also alter, thus reducing the secretions of oils from the sebaceous glands to the skin. These physiological changes are inevitable and irreversible. But while we cannot prevent the ageing, we can slow down this process.

Slowing down the ageing process

Dry skin is one of the most obvious manifestations of ageing skin but we can, by following a number of procedures, take positive steps to increase the skin's moisture. The important thing is to get into the habit of moisturising regularly; the earlier in life you develop this routine the better, but even an older, neglected skin will noticeably benefit from frequent moisturising. No product can really *add* moisture to the skin, despite the claims of some cosmetics manufacturers — all it can do is try to prevent the skin from losing the natural moisture it has already.

The most effective moisturisers are water in oil emulsions, often sold as cold creams or barrier creams. Petroleum jelly is especially effective although most women find it too sticky, but there are many other, more absorbent moisturisers. In searching for the one that suits you best, remember that perfumes and additives can irritate some skins, that creams specially designed for 'dry or ageing' skins are probably no better than any other and that, whatever your age, you do not need to spend a great deal of money on moisturisers with 'magical' ingredients.

Tips for dry and ageing skins

1 Moisturise the skin regularly, paying particular attention to the rough skin on elbows, knees and feet.
2 Use bath oil as an easy way to moisturise your whole body; avoid excessive use of bubble baths and soap which dry the skin.
3 Take neither very hot nor long baths; both destroy natural oils and moisture.
4 Add cream to the hands after doing kitchen chores or wear rubber gloves.
5 Use extra moisturiser or protective creams in windy or sunny weather or when playing sport outdoors.

Tell-tale signs of wrinkles and lines

Nothing shows our age so much as the lines and wrinkles that begin to appear, all too visibly, in early middle age. These first become noticeable around the eyes where the skin is not only at its thinnest but also most affected by facial expression. If you frown a lot, frown lines will appear on your brow; habitual squinting leads to crow's feet; and if you smile a lot you will develop smile lines. As one cosmetic surgeon has observed, '...It's the most expressive areas of the face — the eyes and mouth, for example — that line much more rapidly than the less expressive areas such as the cheeks...we have to pay a price for our active and expressive faces and the price is a skin that ages and lines much more rapidly on the face than it does on the rest of the body.'

The problem is that the muscles on the face are attached directly to the skin, unlike those on the rest of the body which are joined to ligaments or bones. When we exercise these muscles by smiling, frowning, talking and so on, the skin stretches and in a relatively short time begins to wrinkle.

Short-term 'rejuvenation'

There are, however, a few simple treatments that can give an ageing, wrinkled skin some temporary youthfulness. Face masks are the most common. Rinse-off masks are better cleansers but the peel-off ones, which usually contain rubber, wax or some kind of plastic, tighten the skin as they harden. When the mask is peeled off, the blood vessels expand giving the skin a plumper, rosier look and temporarily free of superficial wrinkles.

Another procedure is the removal of dead surface cells. These often accumulate, forming a thick, coarse, leathery outer layer and can be removed with a thinning or abrasive product. With young skin, a rough face-cloth wrung out in warm water will do the trick, but older skin requires heavier treatment. Use a preparation with visible abrasive ingredients like grains (ordinary salt sprinkled on a wet face cloth is a method easy to hand but is not recommended for delicate skin) and rub into the face immediately after cleansing; then rinse off. The thinned skin will look smoother and more translucent and will have a more uniform colour tone. Some, but by no means all, of the fine lines and wrinkles on the face may disappear for a time.

The surgical solution

Plastic surgery is not the answer to *all* the effects of ageing on the skin but it is the only treatment that really can take up to 10 years off your age. It can restore confidence but there are physical, psychological and financial complications

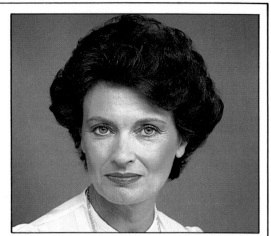

Try colouring your hair naturally in order to disguise grey hairs, and have it set regularly in a soft, flattering style.

that accompany it.

If you are seriously considering cosmetic surgery, it is absolutely essential that you go to a qualified, reputable plastic surgeon. As one surgeon has pointed out, plastic surgery is a branch of medicine, not cosmetic science, and it must be carried out by experts if the risks are to be minimised. Never go to beauty clinics that advertise unless you are absolutely certain that they have suitably qualified surgeons.

The eyes

Blepheroplasty, or eyelid surgery, is one of the most popular and most effective surgical operations. Heavy hoods over upper or lower eyelids and deep lines and wrinkles around the eyes can be corrected by an operation in which a section of the skin and fat is removed and the scar line from the incision either buried a millimetre above the eyebrow or along the edge of the upper or lower eyelid. The operation can be done in about one and a half hours under a local or general anaesthetic, the stitches come out after just three days and the patient will have black eyes or discolouration for up to three or four weeks. Beneficial effects last for up to 10 years.

Face lift for sagging cheeks and jaws

The standard face lift achieves exactly what its name implies. It is a major surgical operation which takes up to three or four hours and requires the patient to be fit and in good health. Using either a general or strong local anaesthetic the surgeon makes small incisions in front of the ears, lifts the skin free from the face and literally pulls it tight before cutting off the excess. The patient needs to spend three to five days in hospital but recuperation tends to be quick with the first stitches coming out after about four days and the last after ten.

Post-operative swelling, bruising and numbness will subside after two or three weeks. Although complications are rare (the official international figure is three per cent), excessive bleeding and infection can occur. More important, a misjudgement during the operation (very rare) can result in the severance of a major nerve which could leave the patient with permanent paralysis. On the plus side, the operation will subtract between five to seven years from the look of your face.

Hints on cosmetic surgery

1 Decide what you want changed before you visit your doctor or plastic surgeon; at the same time, find out if there is any history of disease in your family.

2 Seek the advice/services of a reputable, qualified plastic surgeon. Do *not* go to clinics that advertise.

3 Avoid over-inflated notions about what cosmetic surgery can do for you. It cannot transform you into a youthful goddess nor change your life.

4 Avoid cheap 'mini face lifts'; these are often offered as 20-minute face 'tucks' either along the forehead or cheeks. Alas, the tucks do not hold and in a short time the face relapses with only the scars to show for it.

Exercise and stay young

An important Russian experiment carried out some time ago took a group of 60-year-olds and put them through a tough physical exercise programme once a week. Ten years later, at the age of 70, they were, on all physiological tests, actually younger.

Of course, life-long exercise is desirable if one wants to maintain a youthful figure into middle-age. But the body is remarkably flexible and responsive and even if you have never exercised much, you can get your body into trim at any age, as the above experiment has shown. If you are out of condition, taking up vigorous exercise suddenly can be harmful. Start gradually and with more gentle regimes. A good way to begin is by walking more — up to an hour a day; do muscle-tightening exercises in the bath or while sitting at a desk or in the car; walk up stairs instead of using a lift or excalator. When you are fit you should carry out more vigorous exercises for a short period each day. Although it is probably not advisable to take up a strenuous sport like squash in middle age, any active sport that you can do at your own speed such as swimming, tennis, golf, and bicycling, is enjoyable.

There is considerable medical evidence on the health benefits to be gained by ordinary exercise. Maintaining muscular strength by exercise keeps the heart muscles and arteries fit; lack of exercise is one of the major contributory factors in the premature degeneration of the blood system and the heart.

Weight and ageing

As we age our metabolic rate slows down (by about five per cent per decade from 20 onwards) and this is why we need less food as we grow older. This fact is often not appreciated by women (and men) who declare, no doubt correctly, that their eating habits have not changed over the decades yet they are much heavier than in their twenties.

There is an old adage that 'men run to tum and women to bum', and this has been scientically confirmed by measuring the thickness of fat at different sites in men and women of different ages. Women usually have more fat around the buttocks and upper thighs. But while they may not have much control over *where* their fat is deposited, they can certainly control the amount of fat.

Quite apart from the health risks of being overweight you will look and feel much younger if you keep your weight down. There is really no need for any woman to be more than 4-5kg/8-10lb heavier than she was, say, in her late twenties. Starvation and crash diets are not a good idea as these shrivel the body and collapse the face of middle-aged women, but any well-balanced slimming diet that suits your tastes and way of life will help you slim down. Thereafter, only a little effort is required to maintain that weight. Keep a careful eye on the scales and weigh yourself at least once a week;

you will find it much easier to take off a couple of pounds at a time rather than a stone of fat. For middle-aged women an intake of no more than 1800 calories a day will probably maintain your weight.

Beauty tips for older women

Thirties

1 This is when weight problems begin to appear, especially among women who are still producing children. Watch your weight carefully during and after pregnancy; give yourself and your family *healthy* food. Weigh youself at least once a week and cut back as soon as the scales register two or three pounds extra.

2 Do try to keep up the active sports you played in your twenties, or take up some exercise regime that suits your lifestyle (many women find that yoga not only maintains fitness but provides relaxation from the stresses and strains of family life). If you are having babies, make sure you follow recommended pre- and antenatal exercises.

3 Cleanse and moisturise your skin daily. Don't stay in the bath too long and always add *oil*. Keep out of the sun or take protective measures against it.If you work or live in an air-conditioned/centrally heated environment ensure that the air does not become too dry.

Forties

1 It is even more important to watch your weight now than in your thirties: (a) because your metabolic rate is slowing down and you therefore need less food; and (b) because you are more prone, in your forties, to age and weight-related diseases such as high blood pressure, heart disease and so on.

2 Exercise regularly to tighten up sagging muscles and flesh. If you can, it is both mentally and physically invigorating to take up a sport such as golf or tennis.

3 Take extra special care of the skin by moisturising it regularly. Exfoliate once every couple of weeks and on special occasions use a face mask to tighten and brighten the skin and temporarily get rid of wrinkles. Do try and stay out of the sun.

Fifties

1 With children probably no longer dependent on you, this decade can be one of the most liberating and stimulating of your life, if you make the effort to involve yourself in activites hitherto denied you because of family ties, lack of time etc. Now is the time to embark on hobbies — or even a career — that will interest you for the rest of your life. If your attitude is positive and there is a sense of purpose about what you do, you really will look and feel much younger than your years.

2 This is the time when most women undergo the menopause and it is often accompanied by distressing emotional and physical symptoms. If you experience these, consult your doctor and ask about hormone replacement therapy.

3 Care for your skin and figure much more assiduously than in previous decades since the effects of ageing really begin to show now. Above all, be physically active — it can take years off your shape and skin, and delay age-related diseases.

Sixties

1 The 'age of retirement' should not mean retiring from life — or your job if you can help it. Use your leisure time actively and constructively and stay young.

2 Make sure your diet is healthy and varied and remember that as you grow older you need *less* food; stimulate cell renewal and keep your figure and muscles in trim by regular physical exercise.

3 Have regular medical examinations to check for any signs of debilitating diseases that come with age. If you are listless and tired, take vitamin/mineral supplements and/or herbal remedies. Try to avoid the use of cortisone, barbiturates, toxic antidepressants and tranquillisers, which can have long-lasting side-effects.

Seventies and after

1 It is especially important now to be as physically active as you can be. It really will keep you looking and feeling young and fit and help ward off the inevitable debilities of old age. Do gentle exercises, walk as much as you can and continue to play golf, bowls or similar sports.

2 Watch your diet and weight. Eat small but *healthy* meals. Do not fall into the habit, common among widowed people, of having pre-packed or frozen 'snack' meals because you feel it is not worth cooking for one. Eat fresh fruit, vegetables, fish meat and poultry *regularly*.

3 Take vitamin supplements; they can do nothing but good.

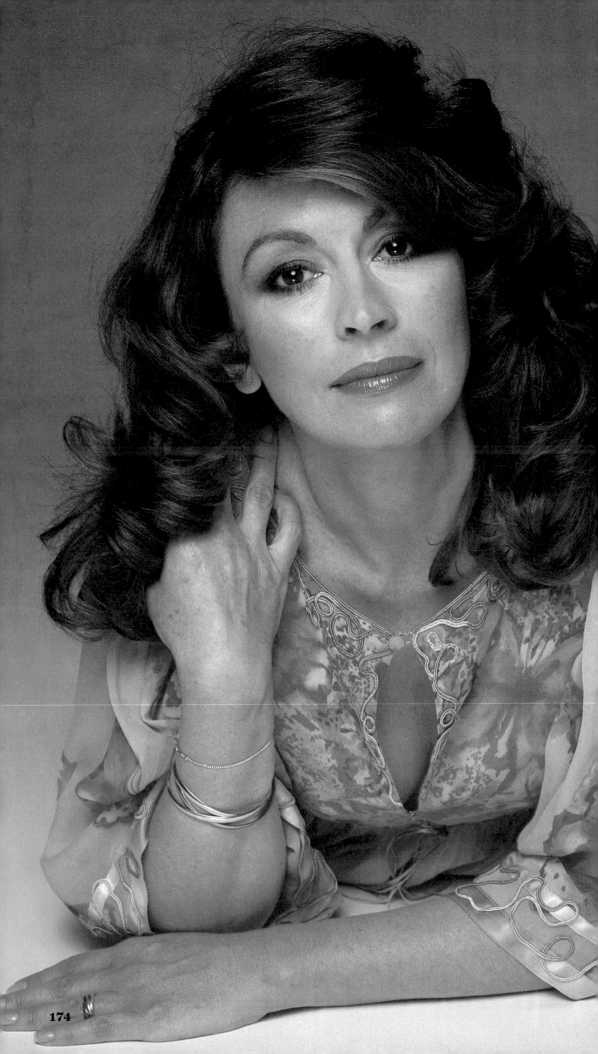

HEALTH & BEAUTY PROFILE

Nanette Newman

Actress Nanette Newman finds time to enjoy a healthy lifestyle despite her busy working schedule. Although she has two grown up daughters she always looks incredibly youthful and beautiful. She says, "We live in an age where everybody is obsessed with age and the best way to stay young is not to have it uppermost in your mind all the time. I don't have any kind of set routine or rules as I lead a very chaotic life, my work takes me abroad a lot and everything I do has to have a rather erratic plan. I manage to convince my self that being busy is one of the best ways of staying healthy!"

Nanette enjoys entertaining and loves to cook, but she always tries to plan healthy meals for her family and guests. "I think that people are eating more healthily nowadays and they're glad to be given a really healthy dinner. At home we never have white sugar, white bread or white flour. I very rarely use anything out of a tin. I always try to cook with fresh ingredients as so much food is adulterated now and I think we're killing ourselves with what we eat."

"I try not to over-eat and diet in fits and starts. I think the best thing to do is to eat sensibly for as much of the year as you can as it's your basic day-to-day diet that counts. I usually have coffee and an apple for breakfast, salad or fruit for lunch, and a meal in the evening. I try to eat just one main meal a day but sometimes I weaken and have a disaster day. I feel better and have more energy when I eat less. I eat a lot of fish but not much red meat as I get very worried about what they're doing to animals and chickens nowadays. We have all been brought up on the habit of meat and two vegetables and a Sunday roast, and it is difficult to break away from this. It takes more thought to cook meals without meat but it is possible, especially in the summer when you can eat more salads."

Nanette thinks that you should not feel guilty if you have days when you over-eat or are tempted by chocolate cakes and other unhealthy foods. "You have to go out and enjoy other things. It's silly to become fanatical about food."

Although she does not exercise regularly, Nanette admits that she does feel better when she manages to find time for it. Leading such a busy life, it is often difficult to fit in any physical activity or sport on a regular basis. "I go through periods when I suddenly exercise every day. I do it when the mood takes me, often when I'm watching television in the evening. I'm sure that if you can bring yourself to exercise regularly you do feel good."

You could be forgiven for thinking that Nanette spends a lot of time on her appearance, especially for a television show, but she has, in fact, got her beauty routine down to a fine art which takes her the minimum possible time. She can wash her hair, get changed and ready to go out in 30 minutes — even faster than it takes her husband to get ready! "Cleanliness is very important and a great thing for skin and hair. Keeping your skin clean is vital and I would not dream of going to bed without cleansing first to remove all my make-up. I wash my hair often as I hate the feel of dirty hair. It depresses me. When it's clean you feel so much better. And I wear as little make-up as possible."

To stay healthy, Nanette believes in practising preventive medicine. "Basically, the simpler your beauty routine, the simpler and healthier your food, and the less adulterated things you put into your body, the better you feel. I think you have to do the best you can to remain healthy."

Eyes too narrow or too wide?
Clever use of shadows, liners
and eye pencils can make
them appear larger or smaller.

Brows too heavy? They can be
plucked and trimmed into
a slimmer, flattering shape.

Nose too wide or too heavy?
A darker shade of foundation
cleverly applied on either
side will slim it down.

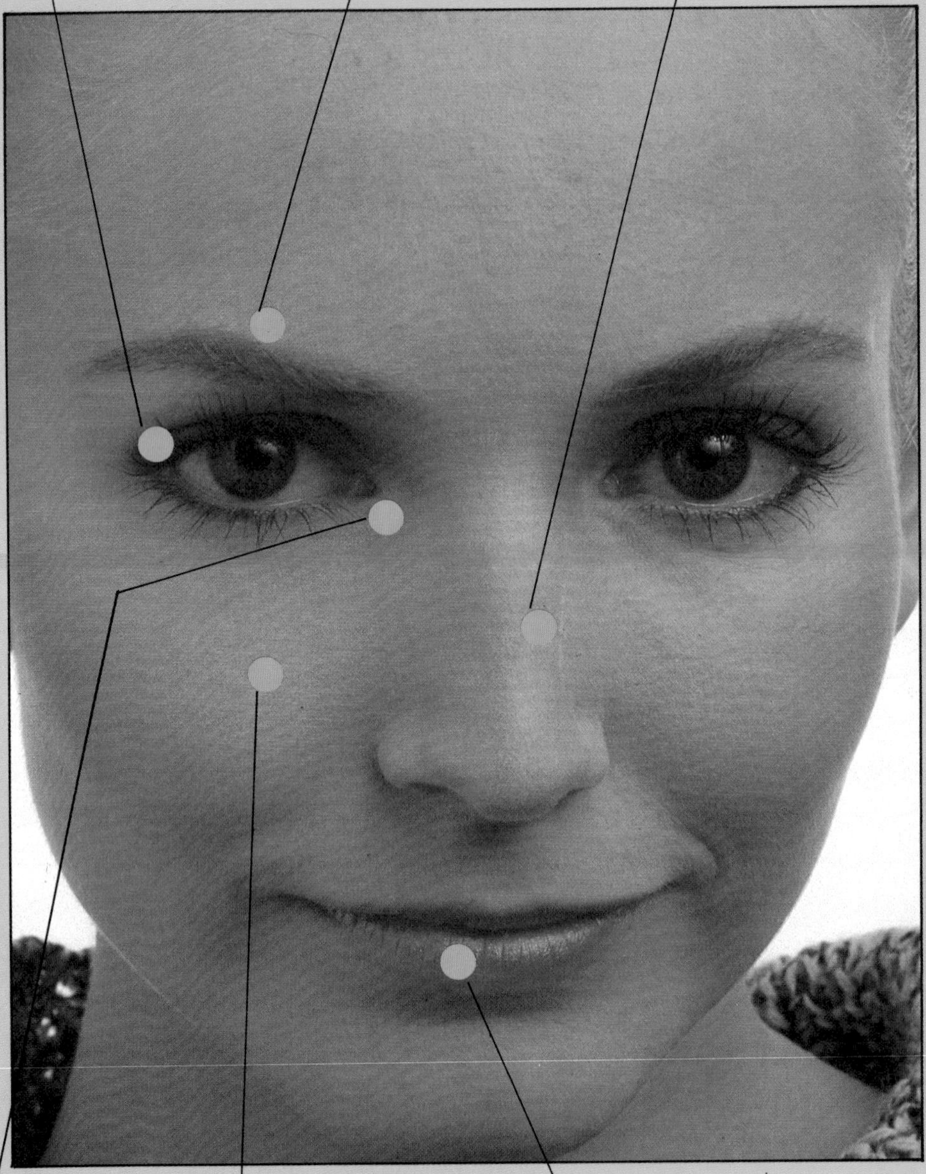

Skin unevenly coloured or too
red? A light matt foundation
evenly applied will make it
appear smooth and uniform.

Lips too full or too thin?
They can be either reduced or
enlarged using different
coloured lipsticks outlined
with a special lip-brush.

Dark shadows under eyes? A
special concealer stick will
disguise them effectively.

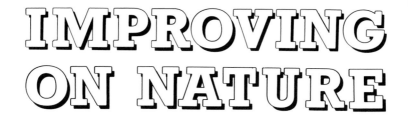

IMPROVING ON NATURE

Now that you are feeling fitter and healthier, you will probably want to show off your glowing skin and all the beauty benefits that your new healthy lifestyle has achieved. You can enhance your new good looks with make-up for a more natural subtle beauty which is more in keeping with your new way of life and the spirit of the 1980s. Today's trend is towards an 'unmade-up' look of subtle understatement, which will make you look younger, healthier and more beautiful. In this way you can make make-up work for you, skilfully enhancing your natural colouring, making the most of your best features and playing down any weak points, such as too long a chin or too thick a nose.

Don't look on make-up as the art of concealment and disguise — a mask that you can hide behind when you come into contact with the ouside world. Rather, it should be creative and fun — a way of reflecting your moods and expressing your own uniqueness. You probably have your own make-up routine which you have used for years and never deviate from, but what was considered fashionable and attractive 10 years ago may not suit you now as styles change and you grow a little older. The secret of good make-up is that it should never look overdone, unnatural or artificial. It is the icing on the cake which makes you feel more confident and attractive as you experiment with different colours and textures to create what looks best for you as an individual.

As well as the usual range of cosmetics, you can also choose from hypoallergenic products which are unscented and specially formulated for delicate, sensitive and allergic skins. Most health food stores sell special ranges of pure cosmetics made from natural ingredients such as plant oils and extracts and containing no chemicals or artificial additives. As a bonus, these cosmetics are tested without cruelty to animals, yet they come in a range of fashionable products and colours.

Before you try out the make-up hints and routine shown here, take a long hard look at your natural unmade-up face. Forget the make-up you usually wear and think about each feature and how you can make the most of it. Consider how shadows, highlights and colour can transform your face in a natural way.

Tools

Good tools — brushes, sponges, sharpeners etc — are essential, as are good light and a large mirror. You will require a selection of different brushes in various sizes for applying blusher, powder, eye shadow, lip colour and highlighters. Keep them clean and well washed and leave to dry naturally away from artificial heat. A good sponge is useful for applying foundation really smoothly and evenly. Always wash it out after use. You may also need cotton wool or cotton tipped buds for wiping away smudged mascara and eyeliner and lipstick. Tissues are useful for blotting make-up and lipstick, and always keep some spring water handy in a plant mister or aerosol container for 'setting' your make-up. An ordinary pencil sharpener is suitable for keeping eye, kohl and lip pencils pointed and sharp.

Skin — the foundations

Unless you have really clear unblemished skin with even colouring, you will probably need to wear some form of skin make-up. Not only will it enhance the natural colouring and beauty of your skin, but it will also help moisturise it and protect it against pollutants in the air and the drying effects of wind and sun.

The colour and type of foundation you choose will depend on your skin's natural colouring, type and condition. As a general rule, it should be as near as possible to your natural skin tone so that no glaring differences in colour are apparent between your face and neck, and should provide only a light covering. Whereas fair skins require only a light, pale foundation, darker skins need more earthy tones. Brown and black skins look better with lighter gels in bronze or earthy shades.

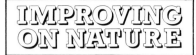
If you have young healthy skin and favour the natural unmade-up look, then a tinted moisturiser which adds glow and light colour is best for you. However, most of us need a matt foundation in cream, liquid, cream and powder base or stick form to give overall colour and texture. Most are beige-pink, beige-rose or more earthy bronze shades. Subtle tones of apricot, gold and peach can also be very flattering, especially for evenings.

Whereas a cream or oil-based liquid are best for dry skins, oily skins will benefit from a water-based foundation which is free from oil. It should be applied sparingly and then powdered lightly to prevent greasy skin shining through. You can apply foundation with your fingertips,

1 Study your naked face in a mirror and try to assess its strong and weak points. Decide which you are going to emphasise and which you should minimise or play down: such as too wide a nose or too strong a jaw.

2 Apply a light even covering of foundation with a damp make-up sponge, taking care to make it appear a uniform shade overall without any streaking or blotches. Be sure to blend it into your neck under your jaw.

dabbing it onto the centre of your face and then smoothing it lightly outwards to give an even overall covering. Take care to blend it well under the chin into the neck so that no dividing line is visible. Or, for a really smooth natural finish, you can use a damp make-up sponge.

For a healthy, sporty look the light tinted moisturising creams and liquids are best although they will not cover blemishes and broken veins. A thicker fluid or cream is needed for this. When choosing a foundation in the store, test a little out on your face, not your hand — the skin tones are quite different.

Cover-ups and concealers

Having applied your foundation you will probably want to disguise any blemishes, scars, spots or birthmarks. For this, you will need a special concealer stick or covering product in the same shade as your foundation so that it can be blended into the colour of the surrounding skin. However, you may need to use a slightly darker product on a livid white scar or a lighter shade on a dark birthmark. Concealers can also be used on dark rings under the eyes, using a light shade and

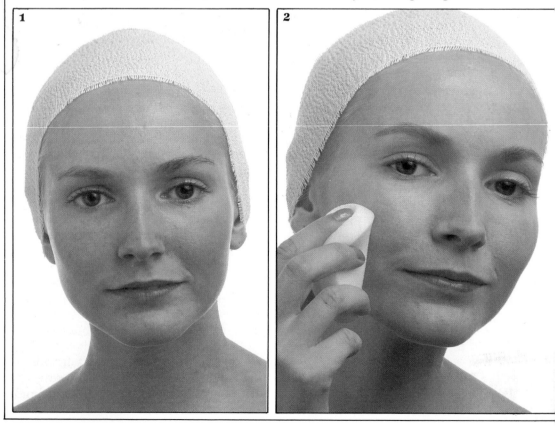

1

2

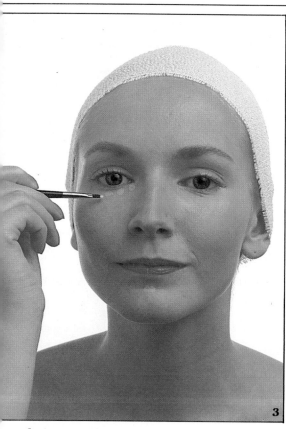

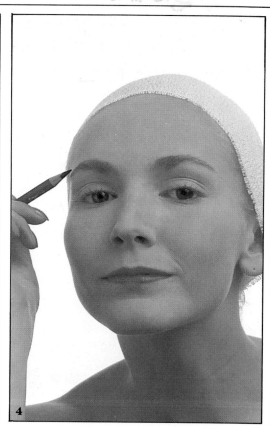

being careful not to harm the delicate and sensitive skin in this area.

Face-shaping and highlighting

You can skilfully contour and highlight your face to change its shape, play up its best features and minimise others such as a wide nose or a heavy jaw. Success depends on the subtle use of light and shade, and heavy-handed attempts will probably do more harm than good. Here are some tips for you to try out:

1 Minimise a large jaw by shading the outer edges with a slightly darker shade of foundation.

2 Disguise a double chin by blending darker foundation into the skin under the chin and gently receding it into the neck.

3 Make a large nose less obvious by shading the sides with a dark foundation.

4 Slim down too round a face by dark shading below each cheekbone.

5 Make a wide bridge at the top of your nose less obvious by applying a darker foundation on either side towards the inner edges of the eyebrows.

Highlights can also play their part, exaggerating high cheekbones, and arching eyebrows to make eyes appear wider. Smooth gently into the small lines running in the hollows from your nose to the edges of the mouth to minimise them.

3 Dot some concealer liquid in the same shade as your foundation under each eye and blend into your make-up to disguise any dark shadows. Use to cover up spots too.

4 Pluck and brush your eye brows into a natural shape. Use an eye-pencil in not too dark a shade to define them in short and gentle strokes. Powder them very lightly and then brush them into shape.

Eyes — making the most of them

Having laid the foundations for your make-up, the next step is to make the most of your eyes. Many women consider them to be their best feature and emphasise them as much as possible, although others strive to make them look larger, smaller, less prominent or deep-set. A natural approach is best for daytime with more dramatic special effects reserved for evenings out.

1 Your eyes will need subtle definition first of all, either with a pencil crayon for a soft smudged effect, or liner for a more definite line. Draw the line close to upper and lower lashes, wiping away any smudges with some cotton wool. You can apply kohl, if wished, on the inner lids.

2 Colour your eyelids with powder, cream, crayons or gels to add shape and interest. The base colours for everyday lie in the grey/brown/green range. Matt, muted colours are best, with frosted shadows and bright pinks and blues, silvers and golds being better suited to evening wear under artificial light. Try experimenting with colours and shading to create new looks, blending different colours into each other. You can either have a darker colour on the lid itself and fade it away into lighter shades near the brow to accentuate and enlarge small eyes, or lighten the lid with a dark crease line to add depth. Powders tend to last longer than creams and gels which may go greasy and smudge as the day wears on.

3 Mascara should be applied last of all, either from a wand or in cake or tablet form. Gradually build up in layers for longer, darker, thicker lashes. Remember to stroke the upper lashes downwards for colour above, before sweeping them upwards for colour below. There is no need to wear a waterproof mascara every day unless you are going swimming or walking in the rain! A gentler product is more suitable for sensitive eyes, is easier to remove and also does not damage surrounding skin or cause wrinkles. And unless you are naturally very dark, choose a brown or greyish mascara in preference to black which can be very harsh. You

can change the shape and size of your eyes with skilful make-up.

Here's a brief basic guide:

1 Make small eyes larger by drawing a fine line close to the lower eyelashes and blending dark shadow outwards from the centre of the lid, leaving the inner lid paler to enlarge the eye.

2 Reduce the impact of large, prominent eyes by smoothing dark shadow across the lid into the crease line with lighter shades above. Kohl on the inner lids will lessen any bulging effect.

3 Make heavy-lidded eyes less obvious by cleverly blending a small triangle of shadow in a medium shade from the centre of the lid into a point on the brow. Highlight the centre of the triangle and draw a smudged crease line at the outer edge.

4 Bring deep-set eyes forwards by using light shadow on the lids with a darker shade above and highlighting the brows.

Your mouth — the expression of you

Your mouth should never be more or less noticeable than your eyes, rather they should balance each other. You eat, drink, communicate and express emotions with your mouth, and it is the most mobile part of your face.

For your new, natural healthy look,

Gently apply some blusher along your cheekbones upwards towards your hairline. Be sure to do it lightly and subtly and not in vivid splashes of bright pink colour.

Outline each eye with pencil along the upper lid close to the lashes and half-way in on the lower lid. Fade and smudge it gently at the corners with a soft-tipped brush.

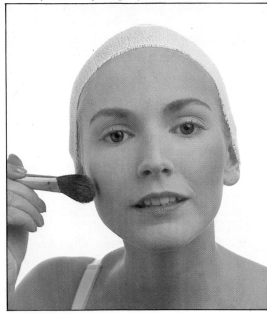

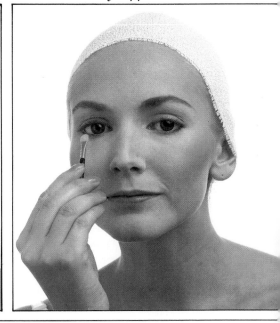

you might like to just apply some gloss for a colourless shine, but coloured lipsticks in muted shades provide more definition and shape. Bright reds, oranges and fuchsia pinks are better suited for evening wear so choose softer pinks, light browns and more earthy shades for daytime. Lipstick will help prevent your lips cracking and drying in winter or burning in summer (when a sunscreen should be worn underneath). Many women apply lipstick badly and it ends up smudged around the mouth. Always use a special fine lip brush to apply colour to the outer edges and outline the shape of your mouth and then fill in with colour. Blot with a tissue and apply a second coat for a longer-lasting effect. In this way you can change the appearance of your mouth also.

1 Thicken thin lips by outlining lightly *outside* your natural lip line, smudge the line softly and then fill in with a darker colour or shade.

2 Make thick lips appear neater and smaller by outlining with a thin brush just *inside* your natural lip line and fill in with a lighter matt shade of lipstick.

3 Equalise lips of different sizes by using a darker shade on the thinner lip and a lighter shade on the thicker one.

The finishing touches

The last touch of all in your make-up routine involves the use of powder and blusher to add colour and finish to your face. A dusting of blusher on your cheekbones will add a healthy glow. Apply it very lightly along the bones themselves towards the hair line and *not* across the whole cheek. Go for a subtle rose, peachy or copper tone which is only a shade or two darker than your foundation and will merge naturally into the surrounding skin colour. It should not stand out unnaturally as a bright spot of colour on either side of a pale face! Pearlised gold and silver blushers are best for evening wear. Creams, gels and powders are available, although powders are most suitable for slightly oily skin and tend to last longer and smudge less. You can add blushers after the foundation stage if wished.

The trend now is to use colourless translucent powder to give your face that finished look and make your skin look younger and smoother. It is particularly effective on oily skins as it eliminates shine. Dust lightly with loose powder, brushing off any excess with cotton wool so that it forms an invisible protective barrier between your skin and the atmosphere. If your make-up needs a quick repair job later on that day, apply pressed powder lighlty.

Finally, you can 'set' your make-up by spraying gently with a fine film of spring water, either from a pressurised container or even a plant mister.

Now apply some eye shadow in a soft shade, such as a muted pink or brown, making it deeper on the lids themselves and then fading it out and upwards towards the brows.

Outline your lips with a very fine brush and carefully fill them in with lipstick in a soft, muted shade. Pat lightly with a tissue and then apply another coating of colour.

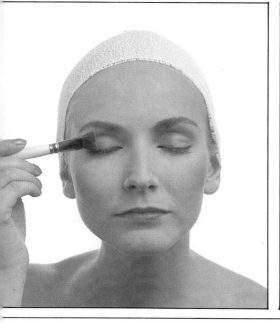

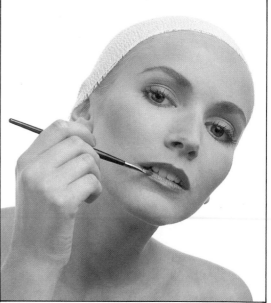

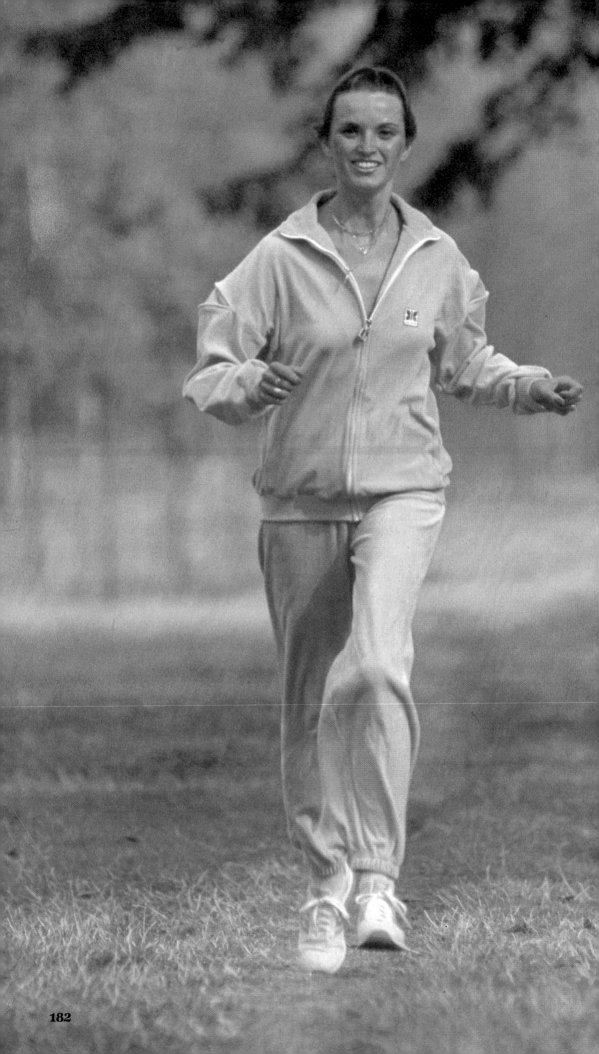

Helen Campbell-Ede

''I've always exercised and tried to keep fit and slim'', says Helen Campbell-Ede, a dentist with a busy practice in London's West End. Now she is training hard to run a marathon although she only started running seriously less than a year ago. Under the supervision of top marathon runners Ian Thompson and Leslie Watson, she volunteered with other 'guinea pigs' who wanted to complete a marathon course (26 miles and 385 yards). She trains between 30 and 40 miles every week, usually in the evenings after work.

It was tough when she first started, walking and running alternately for 15 minutes at a time, but now she is fitter, she finds it much easier. ''I always enjoy the first couple of miles which are more of a warm-up, but then I start to concentrate on my running. I always feel good afterwards and feel that I have really achieved something. I wanted a form of exercise that would fit into my busy lifestyle. Apart from my dental practice, we socialise a lot and my husband's work means that we have to travel most weekends. Running is ideal because I can take my shoes and shorts with me.''

Helen thinks that although she tends to eat more now that she runs regularly, running does help control her weight. ''Whenever the pounds started piling on in the past, I would always exercise or go out for a jog. I used to go swimming, ice skating and play a lot of tennis. I also walk a lot. I walk to work every day and home again in the evening. I make a conscious effort to exercise every day. I always do 20 sit-ups and knee-bends in the mornings, and try to work-out for 20 minutes on my exercise bike.''

''By getting fitter, you feel and look better. I used to get very tired at the end of a day at work, but now I am full of energy and have more vitality. Running has helped me to sleep better and to feel more relaxed. It's also a good outlet for stress which can be quite high in my job. I think that 30 minutes' aerobic exercise, three times a week, raises your metabolism and helps keep you fit and slim.''

Helen is health-conscious about her diet and tries to eat natural foods although she admits to having a weakness for sweets and chocolates and has to ration herself. ''My golden rule is to eat a little of everything in moderation. It's better to have a little of what you want than to try and cut it out completely. If I eat a big evening meal I can compensate by eating less the next day or burn it off by going out for a run. I think that most naturally slim people tend to eat in moderation and are also naturally active. I have very little breakfast — just a coffee and a chocolate biscuit. I have a light lunch — a piece of cheese or a prawn cocktail. I usually eat my main meal in the evening. I rarely eat meat but I love fish and shellfish. I like vegetables, salad and fruit, and I naver eat fried foods. I don't eat cake and I never have sugar in tea or coffee. The only bread I eat is wholemeal.''

Helen thinks that a lot of women worry needlessly about losing their femininity when they take up an active sport. ''A lot of sportswomen, especially in athletics, do look unattracive but this needn't happen to you. It's important to me that I should look good and well-groomed even when I go out running. It gives me confidence and helps me to run better. I don't consider it a vanity — it's just making the most of your own potential. and when you're running and people smile and say 'hello' it gives you a high and you immediately feel better.''

The 14-Day Health and Beauty Programme

Following this 14-day programme, with its simple day-by-day diary will put you on the right road to establishing new dietary, exercise, relaxation and beauty habits which will become an intergral part of your lifestyle and make you feel healthier and fitter. There are body maintenance (skincare, bathing and haircare) programmes too, and at the end of the fortnight you should feel better and more energetic with increased health and vitality. The basic programme can be adapted to suit your daily routine, whether you are busy at home or at work, married or single — it makes no difference. Just follow the basic diet, introduce some physical activity and perform the exercises for increased flexibility. You will be surprised at the difference it makes and at how much better you will feel and look.

The diet is aimed at teaching you new healthy eating habits rather than at weight reduction. However, you may well find that you lose a couple of pounds or more if you normally eat a lot of sugary, fatty and refined foods. It combines natural wholefood ingredients — fresh meat, fish, poultry, dairy products, vegetables, fruit, cereals and high-fibre foods. Use it as a general framework for healthy eating when the 14 days are over. It is nutritionally well-balanced and need not be more expensive than your usual shopping basket.

In addition to the sports, activities and exercises outlined in the programme, you should incorporate the following exercises into your everyday routine, choosing a time of day that suits you best. These include 10 sit-ups and standing straight and stretching up with your arms raised high above your head as far as you can go, so that you feel the stretch right through your body.

Diet

Here is the basic diet for you to follow. It is reasonably flexible and allows you a degree of choice in what you eat at each meal. If you go out to work, you can prepare a packed lunch along the guidelines given, either the night before or in the morning before you leave home. Store in a sealed container.

Breakfast

Choose one of the following:
1 150ml/¼pint unsweetened natural yoghurt or live yoghurt mixed with sliced fresh fruit, bran and wheat germ.
2 50g/2oz unsweetened muesli served with a little milk and sliced fresh fruit.
3 One egg, boiled, poached or scrambled, served with one slice wholemeal or granary bread/toast with scraping of margarine.

Plus one of the following:
1 One glass unsweetened fruit/vegetable juice.
2 One glass hot water mixed with freshly squeezed juice of ½ lemon.
Plus one of the following:
1 One cup herbal tea.
2 One cup unsweetened tea or decaffeinated coffee.
Plus brewers yeast in tablet or powdered form and vitamin pills if you wish.

Lunch

Choose one of the following:
1 One slice wholemeal or granary bread.
2 Small portion boiled brown rice.
Plus 50g/2oz fish, lean meat, poultry (grilled) or cheese with unlimited salad (lettuce, watercress, Chinese leaves, chicory, endive, spinach, cucumber, celery, raw carrot, tomatoes, peppers, radish, onion, bean sprouts, raw mushrooms, cauliflower florets, courgettes) served with yoghurt dressing.
Plus 1 fruit.
Plus one of the following:
1 One cup of herbal tea.
2 One cup of unsweetened tea or decaffeinated coffee.

Dinner

Choose one of the following:
1 50g/2oz grilled fish, lean meat, poultry or cheese.
2 Omelette made with 2 eggs and tiny knob of butter, flavoured with herbs, tomato, mushroom, seafood etc.
Plus one of the following:
1 Small portion boiled brown rice.
2 Small baked potato in skin served with yoghurt and chives.
Plus one of the following:
1 Unlimited salad as at lunch.
2 Steamed vegetables of your choice.
Plus one of the following:
1 Fresh fruit.
2 Natural unsweetened or live fruit yoghurt.
3 Small piece cheese with celery.
Plus one of the following:
1 One cup herbal tea.
2 One cup unsweetened tea or decaffeinated coffee.

Snacks and drinks

The following can be eaten/drunk freely throughout the day:
1 Mineral water.
2 Sunflower, sesame or pumpkin seeds.
3 Raw vegetables (carrots, celery, peppers).
4 Fruit (apples, citrus fruit, pears, berry fruits, apricots).

Day 1

Start the first day of your programme by making some resolutions to last through at least the duration of the fortnight, if not beyond. No more cigarettes or alcohol and refined foods and sugar. You will have to cut out sweets, chocolates, cakes, biscuits, and sugar to sweeten your tea and coffee. Tell yourself now that you *can* do it.

Make a decision to build some walking into every day of the programme. For example, walk to work instead of bussing or taking the car. Or get off the bus a couple of stops before your usual destination and walk the remaining distance. Or park the car a few blocks away.

Weigh yourself on some accurate scales and record your weight. It will be fun referring back after 14 days on the programme to see if you have lost any weight. Then stand naked in front of a full-length mirror and look critically at your figure. Thighs too bulky and heavy? Waist too thick? Good diet and exercise will help attack and tone up these trouble-spots.

This first day of the programme is gentle and

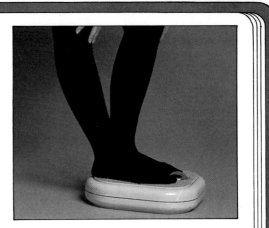

easy. Just start your new diet, do the given exercises, go for a walk, and stay in in the evening and treat your skin to a face pack — try clay if you have oily skin; a peel-off mask if you have dry or normal skin. Don't forget to apply it to your neck too. Remove and moisturise. Now wash your hair and use a deep-action conditioner to restore it to first-class condition. Then curl up in bed with a book and get a good night's sleep.

Day 2

Inspect your skin. Cleanse well, wait at least 10 minutes and then study it at close-quarters in a magnifying mirror. Is it too dry or too oily? Write moisturiser at the top of your shopping list if it is too dry and start working on it now before it becomes lined or wrinkled. Oily skin with spots, whiteheads or blackheads will improve as a result of your new eating habits. But make sure you cleanse it thoroughly with mild foaming cleanser and then freshen and use an oil-in-water moisturiser. This skin routine — cleanse, freshen, moisturise — will last you a life-time.

Give your body an overall conditioning work-out with the work-out programme (see pages 94-109). It only takes 30 minutes, either first thing in the morning, in your lunch-hour or in the evening. Or, if you prefer, you can buy an exercise tape or video — there are lots of good ones to choose from. If you prefer to have the moral support of others, you should enrol today at your local work-out class or studio for a whole course. Start now and make it an unbreakable habit.

If you are working-out at home, wear something comfortable, preferably tights and leotard, and find a warm place with plenty of room to stretch out in all directions. Put on a tape or record with a strong rhythmic beat and start your work-out with a warm-up and some aerobics. Work your way through the exercises for arms and shoulders, waists, stomach, hips and legs and buttocks. Finish with the warm-down and then have a refreshing shower or bath. It will be hard at first and your body will ache a little, but you

will feel good afterwards — invigorated and full of energy!

Buy some dental floss and use it before you go to bed after cleaning your teeth. Break off a length and, winding each end around the first two fingers of each hand, slide it up and down between your teeth to remove food particles and plaque. Use it at least every day if you want to keep your teeth healthy.

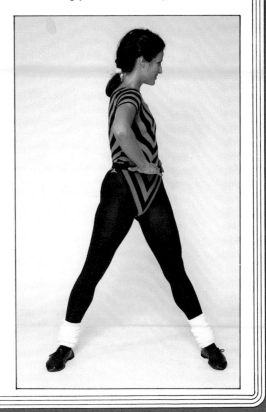

Day 3

Make time today to get out in the fresh air and go for a gentle jog. Wear a tracksuit if you have one, or improvise with shorts or loose trousers and T-shirt or sweatshirt. A pair of running shoes is a worthwhile investment — there are many fashionable styles and you can wear them with jeans or shorts for leisure wear and on holiday. Warm-up with some stretching exercises before you set out. This is very important for warming up your muscles and increasing your heart rate to pump more oxygen around your body as you run. Now step out of the front door and off you go. Nothing could be easier — just run relaxed and breathe deeply and easily. Don't punch the air or hold your shoulders tight and tense. Be natural and un-self-conscious and just enjoy it. If you feel breathless, then slow down and walk a little way until the feeling passes and then start running again. Keep going for 10 minutes and then turn round and run/walk back. Before you collapse into a bath or shower, stretch out your muscles and warm down to combat stiffness.

Relaxation as well as exercise is on the menu for today, so put aside 30 minutes to be quiet and on your own, preferably later in the day after you have eaten, put the children to bed or cleaned up. Instead of just collapsing in a chair in front of the television, try some positive relaxation to alleviate the stress and tension of a busy day. Breathing is very important so lie flat on a level surface with your arms at your sides, palms upwards. Breathe in deeply and slowly all the way down to your abdomen until your lungs are fully expanded. Hold it and count to five slowly. Now gradually exhale

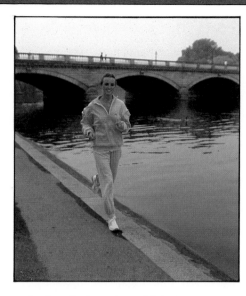

and relax. Do it again and this time put your hands on your abdomen so that you can feel it rise when you inhale, and sink when you exhale.

Now for a little meditation: in the same position, slowly relax your whole body, starting with your facial muscles and neck and shoulders and working down through your chest, arms, hands, abdomen, hips, legs and feet. You should now be completely relaxed. Empty your mind of all thoughts and let it go blank or, if this is too difficult, concentrate on one object only and shut out everything else. After 10 minutes or so, slowly regain control, working upwards from feet to head. Now slowly stretch out as far as you can go, feet in one direction and arms in the other. Relax. You should feel less tense.

Day 4

You may feel a little stiff after your work-out of Day 2 and yesterday's jogging, so walk briskly for one hour today or go for a long cycle. Cycling is good aerobic exercise and will build up cardiovascular fitness and stamina if practised regularly — three or four times a week. Make sure that your bike is in good working order before you set out — tyres are blown up to the correct air pressure, brakes work efficiently, and saddle and handle-bars are adjusted to the right height.

When you return have a special bath and add some fragrant oil to the warm water — choose from basil, citron, lavender, rosemary, jasmine or rose — or you can make a *bouquet garni* of fresh herbs to immerse in the water. Just tie some up in a piece of muslin or cheesecloth and pop in the bath. Now get to work on your body, attacking patches of rough skin on feet, knees and elbows with a loofah or hemp massage mit. Alternatively, squeeze some fresh lemon juice onto these problem areas and rub

away. If you have a massage glove, especially the sort which encloses a bar of specially formulated soap, attack your waist, hips and thighs until they glow.

While you are in the bath, try some special exercises to help tone you up.
1 To firm stomach muscles, sit in the bath with your legs stretched out in front of you. Support yourself with your arms held straight out behind you. Now slowly raise yourself on your arms, lifting your buttocks off the floor of the bath. Feel the pull in your stomach muscles. Hold to a count of five and slowly lower yourself again. Repeat 10 times.
2 Now sit up straight with your arms raised high above your head, your legs straight out in front of you. Slowly lift one leg out of the water, as high as you can. Lower, and lift the other leg. Repeat 15 times, keeping your arms raised.

After your bath, pamper yourself and gently rub in some moisturising scented cream or oil to keep skin soft and supple and prevent it getting too dry.

Day 5

Run through your work-out programme, either at home or at a local class. Have a bath or shower. Then do some extra work on your face and neck muscles with some simple exercises. Start by attacking a double chin and firming up that under-chin area generally.

1 Stretch your head back as far as it will go. Feel the stretch in your neck under your chin. Now, to increase the stretch, purse your lips and literally 'kiss' the ceiling. Lower your head and repeat 10 times.

2 Gently but firmly stroke your neck with the fingers of both hands upwards from the collar bone to your chin. Repeat 10 times.

3 Open your mouth and eyes as wide as you can and hold to a count of five. Relax and repeat 10 times.

Now for some exercises which are beneficial to your eyes and keep the muscles in the surrounding skin firm. If practised regularly, they will help protect you against premature age-lines and wrinkles.

1 Slowly roll your eyes in complete circles, 10 times to the left and 10 times to the right.

2 Hold your forefinger or a pencil about 25-30cm/10-12in in front of your face and focus on it. Now look beyond it to some distant landmark or object for a few seconds and then back to your finger or pencil. You should not move your head, only your eyes. Repeat 10 times.

For todays's beauty treatment, give yourself a facial sauna to stimulate circulation, open pores, eliminate impurities and leave skin glowing and fresh-looking. Place some fresh herbs of your choice in a large basin — try sage or comfrey for sensitive, delicate skin; rosemary, mint or basil for oily skin; or lavender, rose petals and strawberry leaf for normal skin. Fill the bowl (not right up to the brim for safety's sake) with boiling water, and carefully lean over it for 10 minutes with a towel draped over your head, steaming your face. Now splash with cold water and moisturise. Your skin will be really fresh.

Day 6

Go for a swim in the local pool. In addition to being a good form of aerobic exercise, it is great for muscle-toning and firming. Practised regularly, it will reshape and streamline your body, particularly if you are a little over-weight. You need to swim for at least 15 minutes without stopping to receive any real benefits. However, it will probably seem easier than running or cycling because the water supports your body as you move along. Choose a time of day when the pool is not too crowded and you can swim backwards and forwards without interruption.If you dislike swimming or there is no nearby pool, then walk briskly or cycle for 45 - 60 minutes.

Now to combine some relaxation with exercise and stretch out tired muscles, try the following basic yoga asanas (postures).

1 Sunrise stretch: lie face downwards on the floor, your forehead resting on the floor and your hands, palms down, directly under your shoulders. Using your back muscles only, slowly lift your head and shoulders so that you are facing forwards, Inhale deeply and hold for a count of five. Exhale. Now, using your arm muscles only, slowly lift your head and neck as far as they will go and lift your pelvis off the floor, supporting your weight with your hands and feet. Inhale and hold for a count of 10. Exhale and then slowly withdraw from the posture and relax. Repeat three times. This is a good overall stretch which loosens the lower back and helps promote good breathing. It will strengthen your spine and lower back muscles, wrists and triceps.

2 Half forward bend: sit up straight with one leg extended in front of you, the other bent beneath you so that your left foot is tucked underneath your right thigh, with your heel resting in your groin. Breathe in deeply and raise your arms above your head. Slowly bend forwards lowering your arms and chest over your outstretched leg until your chin rests on your knee (if you can lower it that far — may take practice). Exhale and grasp your foot between your hands and hold the stretch for a count of 20 if possible, breathing deeply. With practice, as you become more flexible, you will be able to close the space between your thigh and chest. Repeat three times. You will feel the stretch in your hamstrings and buttocks, as well as your spine.

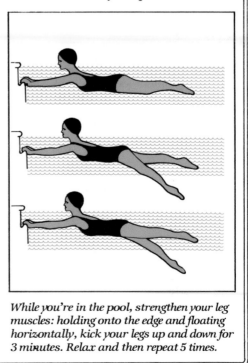

While you're in the pool, strengthen your leg muscles: holding onto the edge and floating horizontally, kick your legs up and down for 3 minutes. Relax and then repeat 5 times.

Day 7

After yesterday's relaxing swimming, it's time for another run, so get changed, warm-up and stretch thoroughly and then run/walk for 20 minutes as you did on Day 3. You will probably find it a little easier today and that you can increase the time you spend running and reduce the periods of walking in between. Don't run flat-out — you are not racing. Just run gently and rhythmically, concentrating on breathing easily and feeling relaxed. After a while, you will probably get your second wind and will feel better — your legs will feel lighter and move more fluidly, your breathing will improve and you will begin to enjoy your run. When you return home, spend 10 minutes warming-down and stretching out your leg muscles, and then bathe or shower.

Check your posture today. Stand in front of a full-length mirror to discover whether you slouch or slump. You will look slimmer and feel better if you stand tall and erect. There will be less strain on muscles and joints and you are less likely to suffer back pain. Practise standing and sitting straight with your stomach pulled in and rib cage lifted up. You can do this in a relaxed way without standing rigidly to attention as though you were being drilled on the parade ground! If you can develop the good posture habit, you will have better digestion and the muscles in your back will be strengthened.

Lastly, give your nails a good manicure and work on your hands to get them into tip-top condition. Spread your hands out in front of you and examine them closely. The skin sould be soft and supple — not chapped, dry, flaky or ingrained with dirt. Your nails should be strong and healthy, smooth and pink — not brittle, weak, dotted with white spots or split. For your home-manicure, you will need some hand-cream, emery boards, orange sticks, some cuticle cream and a bowl of warm water. If your nails are polished you will need some varnish remover and more nail varnish to coat them after the manicure.

1 Remove old nail polish.
2 Shape each nail with an emery board, filing towards the centre.
3 Massage cuticle cream, oil or hand cream around cuticles and soak in warm water. Dry.
4 Ease back each cuticle with an orange stick tipped with cotton wool and soaked in soapy water. Pat dry.
5 Moisturise hands with cream or oil and varnish nails if wished.

Day 8

For today's exercise, walk briskly or cycle for one hour. When you get back, have a shower and give yourself a massage to ease out tension and counteract muscular stiffness. Lie down naked on a flat surface in a warm room. Cover the areas of the body you are not working on with a rug or blanket. The secret of good massage is to move your hands rhythmically and firmly — you do not have to pummel and hurt yourself.
1 Lying on your back, stroke gently upwards from your abdomen to your ribs, using some oil — sunflower, safflower, lavender, apricot.
2 As the rhythm improves, press harder on the upwards stroke. Now knead each arm and

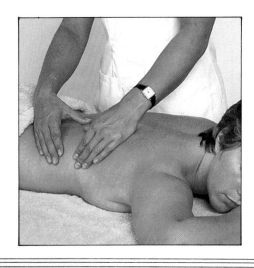

shoulder gently and behind your head at the back of your neck to ease out tension.
3 Massage the backs of your legs, working upwards towards the heart in strong circular movements, paying particular attention to any patches of cellulite on hips and thighs.
4 Ease down by stroking gently and slowly.

As you are half-way through your programme now, treat yourself to a special evening dinner of **Seafood Kebabs**.
You will need the following ingredients for one person (double or treble up as necessary):

175g/6oz firm white fish cut into chunks *or* large prawns *or* scallops
1 small onion, quartered
½ red or green pepper, cut into chunks
2 prunes soaked in water
1 bacon rasher, cut in half
10ml/2 teaspoons oil
juice ½ lemon
chopped fresh herbs
salt and pepper
Thread the fish/shellfish, onion quarters, peppers and prunes wrapped in bacon alternately onto 2 kebab skewers. Mix the oil, lemon juice herbs and seasoning and brush the kebabs. Grill until cooked and faintly browned, basting if necessary.

For **dessert**, make a fruit fool by mixing puréed fresh fruit of your choice (raspberries, strawberries, gooseberries, blackcurrants, apricots etc) with thick yoghurt, and sweeten to taste if wished with honey. *Bon appetit!*

Day 9

Another work-out day so put on a tape and work-out as before or go along to your work-out class. As you become fitter and more familiar with different exercises, the work-out will seem easier and more enjoyable.

Continue waging war on cellulite by drinking two glasses of either carrot, celery, cucumber, apple, watercress or orange juice to flush any toxic wastes out of your system. Keep this up through the remaining days of the programme at least. After your bath or shower, while your skin is warm and receptive, massage any suspect areas on legs and arms.

1 Stroke gently at first, hand over hand.

2 Stroke away from the heart all the time and increase the pressure gradually, kneading firmly and then vigorously to increase the circulation in these 'dead' areas and draw away wastes.

3 Using your knuckles and thumbs, twist into the cellulite in circular movements and then gradually reduce the pressure and stroke again. Use a vegetable oil if wished.

Give your skin a nutritious treat with a yoghurt face-mask.

1 Remove any make-up and cleanse very thoroughly. Pat dry.

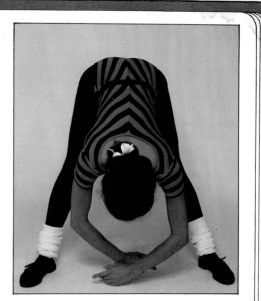

2 Mix together one of the following:
Live natural yoghurt with avocado *or* fresh crushed stawberries and oatmeal *or* brewers yeast powder.

3 Spread the mixture lightly over your face and leave for 20-30 minutes.

4 Rinse off thoroughly and pat dry.

Your skin will look softer and fresher. The avocado mask is excellent for dry skin.

Day 10

For your choice of exercise, you can do one of the following:

1 Swim non-stop for 20 minutes.

2 Walk briskly for one hour.

3 Cycle for about one hour.

Give yourself a home-pedicure. Have ready some nail clippers or scissors, a pumice stone, cuticle cream, and orange sticks.

1 Start if wished by soaking tired, aching feet in a bowl of warm water. You can add Epsom salts if you like.

2 Trim nails with clippers or scissors.

3 Rub a little cuticle cream around the nails and, using an orange stick tipped with cotton wool, ease back the cuticles.

4 Rub away patches of hard skin with a pumice stone or a special liquid remover.

5 Moisturise your feet with cream, and then varnish nails if wished.

Work on your legs to keep them beautiful and in good shape. Here are some special exercises for shaping, firming, improving circulation and reducing musclar tension.

1 Kneel down with your arms extended at shoulder level straight out in front of you, back perfectly straight. Now slowly lean as far back as possible. Hold to a count of five and rise up forwards again. Repeat 10 times.

2 Sit back on your heels with your feet apart and your bottom resting on the floor between them. Put your hands, palms downwards, knees touching eachother, as close to the floor as you can. Hold for a count of 5 and repeat.

3 Lie on your stomach, arms by your sides and very slowly raise your left leg as high as it will go. Hold for a count of 10 and then lower slowly. Raise your right leg and repeat the exercise in the same way. Then raise both legs together. Try to do five repetitions.

Day 11

For a different sort of aerobic exercise, buy a jump-rope and try skipping. You probably haven't skipped since you were a child but it is an excellent all-over conditioner — it improves cardiovascular fitness, burns up calories and strengthens your legs.

It is simplicity itself — all you need is a rope and you can do it anywhere at any time. Practise regularly for at least 20 minutes per session and it will help you get aerobically fit. It burns up about 10 calories per minute. Start off by skipping forwards but as you become more proficient you can vary your skipping by trying a backwards skip and even a cross-over skip. Like other forms of exercise, a warm-up is important so do some gentle stretching exercises before you start to ease out muscles. Stay relaxed while you skip and jump only sufficiently high to just clear the rope each time. Make sure you breathe deeply and regularly and look straight ahead — not at the rope. Wear some running shoes for good shock-absorption when you land.

Give your hair a deep-conditioning treatment, especially if it is dry, dull or with split ends. Just massage some warm almond or olive oil into your scalp. Rub it in well, really working it into the skin. Then wrap up your hair in a

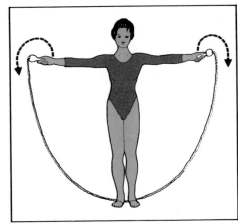

Forwards skip

hot towel (wrung out in hot water) and leave for 20-30 minutes. If the towel starts to cool, wring it out again in hot water so that the oil can do its work. Rinse your hair, shampoo and rinse again to remove all traces of soap. Set in your favourite style and dry in the usual way. Or you could try a temporary colour rinse to add subtle colours and highlights to your hair. It will not damage the hair shafts by stripping away the natural colours, and will last for only one or two shampoos, but it will ring the changes and make you feel different.

Day 12

Work-out in the usual way, either at home or at your local class or exercise studio. If you are feeling fitter and more supple, try introducing some additional repetitions as you go through your exercise routine, say, three to five per exercise. However, stick to the usual number if you feel stiff or tired.

Try a new make-up today — you need not buy some new expensive cosmetic preparations

To strengthen upper arms and tone up flabby areas, practise winding a weight up and down, keeping your arms straight outstretched.

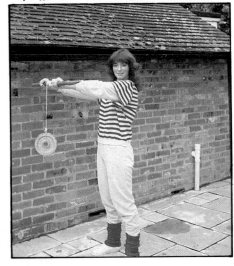

but can experiment with the products you already have by using them differently. Flick through some fashion magazines to get some inspiration and try new ideas out to see what suits you best. It may be that you have got into a make-up rut after using the same look for several years, and what was fashionable then no longer suits you. The new trend is for a more natural look with subtle colours.

Put aside 10 minutes for relaxation and easing tired eyes. After a day at work or outside in sun and wind, eyes may be inflamed and sore. Try one of the following soothing ideas:
1 Splash a few drops of ice-cold witch hazel onto two cotton wool pads and place one over each eye. Lie down for 10 minutes, then remove and rinse your face. Pat dry.
2 Place slices of cold cucumber over each eye and rest for 15 minutes. Rinse and pat dry. Your eyes will look less sore and you will feel refreshed. To freshen tired eyes you can try closing them as tightly as you possibly can, and then open very slowly. Your vision will be clearer and sharper immediately.
Little lines and creases are apt to appear around the corners of eyes from your twenties onwards, especially if you have an expressive face and tend to laugh or scowl a lot. The skin around your eyes is very delicate and has a tendency to be dry, so start a lifetime's good habits now by applying eye cream or oil to the area every night after cleansing. Just gently dab on the bare minimum of cream or a natural oil such as apricot or avocado.

Day 13

Only one more day to go until the end of the programme so set out for your 20 minutes run today with the aim of walking less than usual if at all, and jogging for the full 20 minutes' if you can. Just run relaxed, concentrate on getting your breathing right, don't tense your shoulder muscles but keep them loose and comfortable, and you *can* do it. You will feel a sense of real achievement afterwards at what you have accomplished.

Have a day without meat — just fresh fruit, vegetables, yoghurt, eggs, cheese, grains and cereals. Try a brown rice **pilaff** for your evening meal. Mix freshly cooked vegetables — onions, mushroom, courgettes, asparagus tips and French beans — into some cooked brown rice. Season and sprinkle with grated Parmesan cheese. Serve with salad. You can add a little saffron to the cooking rice and cook it in chicken stock instead of water if wished.

Work-out with weights today to improve muscle tone and get rid of surplus fat. Don't worry about building up unfeminine rippling muscles — this is not possible for most women unless the male hormone testosterone is present in their bodies. Light weights used in repeated repetitions will help firm you up and reduce weight — not add to it with extra muscle bulk. You do not need special dumb-bells — improvise with cans of soup, beer cans or telephone directories.

1 To firm up your bust and chest muscles, lie on your back on the floor with a rug or towel beneath you. Bring up your knees so that they are bent and touching in the middle, with your feet set shoulder-width apart on the floor. Now, with a weight in each hand, inhale and raise the weights above you, keeping your arms straight. Slowly lower your arms out-stretched to the floor on either side of you at right angles to your body, exhaling as you do so. Inhale and raise your arms again, exhale and bend elbows very slightly. Inhale and lower again. Repeat 10 times.

2 To firm up thighs and buttocks, stand with your feet hip-width apart, arms at your sides and a can of soup in each hand. Now bend your legs slightly and inhale deeply as you lower your arms, keeping your back straight. Rise slowly back to the starting position and exhale. Repeat 10 times.

Always stretch out your calf and hamstring muscles before setting out for a run.

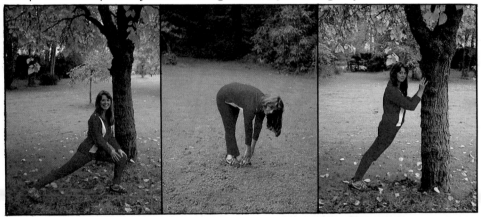

Day 14

Well, you have made it to the end of the programme. Do you feel fitter, slimmer, more supple? Does your skin look healthier, clearer and glowing? Does your hair look glossier and silkier? Weigh yourself and compare the reading with that of your first day. Unless you have cheated, your weight will probably be less or at least the same.

Don't neglect your exercise today — go for a swim, cycle or a brisk walk, and run through your daily exercises. Now write down what you think you have achieved — for example, weight loss, new interests, better dietary habits, a sleeker, more supple body, better skin and a healthier lifestyle. Make some resolutions for the coming weeks and months ahead don't feel smug and abandon your new diet and exercise regime and resume your old bad habits. Adapt it to your usual timetable and find ways of building exercise and good food into your lifestyle. Resist the temptation to smoke another cigarette or celebrate your success with a drink. Instead, buy a new scent, make-up or clothes.

The comprehensive programme incorporated a diet, exercise and beauty treatments that would cost you considerable money to enjoy at a health farm. You have had the discipline and dedication to do it by yourself at home and at work, and it will be easier for you to make these new habits last a lifetime. Continue with the sport or exercise that you enjoy, and even if you cannot resist the occasional chocolate bar or glass of wine, cut down on these indulgences and make up for occasional lapses by eating plenty of natural wholefoods daily. Use the programme as a basis for future healthy living.

Index